WINNING THE BATTLE AGAINST UNWANTED HAIR GROWTH

WINNING THE BATTLE AGAINST UNWANTED HAIR GROWTH

Laura M. Regan

"Books are the quietest and most constant of friends; they are the most accessible and wisest of counselors, and the most patient of teachers." —Charles W. Eliot

Divine Books

WINNING THE BATTLE AGAINST UNWANTED HAIR GROWTH

For further information, please contact:
divinelaser@hotmail.com

Book design by: RECEIVED SEP 0 4 2007

Arbor Books, Inc.
19 Spear Road, Suite 301
Ramsey, NJ 07446
www.arborbooks.com

Printed in the United States

WINNING THE BATTLE AGAINST UNWANTED HAIR GROWTH
Laura M. Regan

1. Title 2. Author 3. Cosmetic Dermatology/Laser Hair Removal

Library of Congress Control Number: 2006907005
ISBN 10: 0-9788341-0-0
ISBN 13: 978-0-9788341-0-0

ACKNOWLEDGEMENTS

First and foremost I want to commend my patients, friends and family members who were brave enough to talk about their conditions so openly and honestly with me. Every story profoundly touched my life. You are my heroes! Thank you for making the past 18 years of research worthwhile!

I am also grateful to Vaniqa®, Skin Medica as well as Palomar Medical Technologies for their continued support, dedication, incredible business knowledge and unparalleled resources. Kahtie—you're the best! Harriet—you may not even remember me but you were the one who introduced me to the world of hair removal which opened the door to a career for me.

This book would not even exist without my extraordinary family. Andy—you are a saint for putting up with me and supporting me so completely over the years. I am so incredibly thankful to you and my three amazing children—Sean, Julia and "Little" Andy. You guys are everything to me.

Thank you also to Mom, Dad, Ali, "Pee-Pa," The McNamara Clan, The Sjolanders, Maryann (Momma Bear), and Ashley.

I am indebted to Dr. Tutera and SottoPelle® and Dr. Tala Dajani.

My final "Thank you" goes out to all of the hard-working, wonderful people at Arbor Books. Great job! A million thanks!

CONTRIBUTORS

I would like to recognize the following companies for their support and contributions. They offered a great amount of information for this book. Their endorsements are also greatly appreciated.

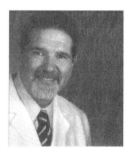

Gino Tutera, M.D., F.A.C.O.G.,
Medical Director, SottoPelle,
www.sottopelletherapy.com
"Without a doubt the book is one of the best resources on the subject of hirsutism and the choices of treatment available."

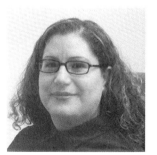

Tala Dajani MD MPH
Pediatric Endocrinologist
Phoenix Children's Hospital
1919 East Thomas Rd
Phoenix, AZ 85016
602.546.0935
602.546.0610 fax
tdajani@phoenixchildrens.com
"This book will give young ladies and women with hirsutism information and resources to deal with this very difficult problem. Regan's enthusiasm and positive attitude comes through. An excellent resource and quite due. Bravo!"

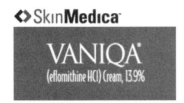

Skin Medica® (Vaniqa®),
SkinMedica, Inc., 5909 Sea Lion Place, Ste H, Carlsbad, CA 92010 USA
www.skinmedica.com

"…very thorough and informative. Great for patients researching which type of therpy is best for them. The book includes impressive detailed descriptions of treatment options available today."

—Richard E. Fitzpatrick, M.D., Founder, Chairman, Scientific Advisory Board, SkinMedica, Inc.

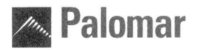

Palomar Medical (IPL—Medilux, Starlux etc.),
82 Cambridge Street, Burlington, MA 01803
www.palmed.com

DISCLAIMER

The information contained in this book is intended to provide helpful health information for the general public. It is made available with the understanding that the author and publisher are not engaged in rendering medical, health, psychological, or any other kind of personal professional services in this book. The information should not be considered complete and does not cover all diseases, ailments, physical conditions or their treatment. It should not be used in place of a call or visit to a medical, health or other competent professional, who should be consulted before adopting any of the suggestions in this book or drawing inferences from it.

Any information about drugs, alternative remedies, and/or therapies contained in this book is general in nature. It does not cover all possible uses, actions, precautions, side effects, or interactions of the medicines mentioned, nor is the information intended as medical advice for individual problems or for making an evaluation as to the risks and benefits of taking a particular drug.

The author and publisher make no warranties or representation as to the effectiveness of the suggestions in this book. The author and publisher specifically disclaim all responsibility for any liability, loss or risk, personal or otherwise, which is incurred as a consequence, directly or indirectly, of the use and application of any of the material in this book.

CONTENTS

INTRODUCTION

EXCESSIVE, UNWANTED FACIAL AND BODY HAIR

Demographics and Statistics

Hirsutism is *abnormal* or male-like pattern hair growth in places where coarse, dark hair is not normally found on a woman (upper lip, chin, sides of face, and neck), as well as parts of the body (nipples, chest, lower arms, upper legs, abdomen, back) as defined by the individual woman according to her personal opinion of acceptability. If a woman feels she has *excessive facial hair,* then she does! This growth is caused by an excess of any of the male hormones called *androgens.* Basically, *hair follicles* are being over-*stimulated* by testosterone or other androgen hormones.

When a *diagnosis* of hirsutism is made, one must rule out the possibility of an underlying medical condition, most commonly *PCOS* (Polycystic Ovarian Syndrome) or *CAH* (Congenital Adrenal Hyperplasia). Androgen-secreting tumors, although rare, must also be ruled out as an etiology. Hirsutism is more commonly referred to as *Unwanted Facial Hair* (UFH) and *Unwanted Body Hair* (UBH).

A woman's definition of hirsutism may differ depending

1

upon her interpretation of *normal,* which is often influenced by popular images of hairless female beauty. Our culture tends to determine how much hair is cosmetically acceptable. Also, any definition of normal body hair must take into consideration race and ethnicity. Most Asian and Native American women have little body hair, while Mediterranean women on average have moderately heavy body hair. However, hirsutism can affect women of ALL nationalities, ethnicities and ages. The most important consideration, whatever the woman's background, is whether the pattern of hair growth has changed or the rate of growth has increased.

Unwanted facial hair (UFH), as well as unwanted body hair (UBH) is not a disease; it is a *condition* (a *chronic* condition). Unwanted hair growth is an extremely sensitive issue which negatively impacts *self-esteem.* UFH and UBH often cause women to feel self-conscious about appearance, and have lasting effects on self-image. The *psychological impact* of "being hairy" can range from annoying to severely *disabling.* As critical as this *condition* is, our society treats the topic as *taboo,* and mainstream America does not discuss it openly. This *vital* issue lacks the attention it so greatly deserves. Women are desperate for answers but are too embarrassed to ask the questions.

Many of the *italicized* words above are not only defined in the glossary in Chapter 20, but also meticulously detailed throughout this book along with anything and everything you need to know about "being hairy" and becoming permanently "not hairy"!

Statistics About Unwanted Facial Hair and Hirsutism:

- In the United States: Hirsutism is common and is estimated to occur in 1 in 20 women of reproductive age.

- Internationally: Familial hirsutism is found most

commonly in southern European and South Asian countries in which it is considered to be a normal trait. Hirsutism indicative of underlying endocrinopathy varies from culture to culture, depending on the incidence of the various endocrinopathies in a particular society.

- Nearly 90 percent of UFH cases are a result of hereditary or physiologic factors related to hormonal changes at puberty or menopause (*only 7 percent are attributed to underlying medical conditions*).

- Nearly *41 million* women have removed unwanted facial hair in the last 6 months.

- 22 million women (1 out of every 5) remove unwanted facial hair *weekly or daily*, or remove at least 20 hairs at a time.

- Only 10 percent of the 22 million women (1 out of every 5 women in the U.S.) who remove UFH weekly or daily consult a doctor about their UFH.

- 8 percent of women rely strictly on the superior technology and expertise of licensed professionals to perform hair removal procedures.

- *Only 4 percent of women discuss their condition with friends or family members.*

- Approximately 70 percent of women with a history of PCOS (Polycystic Ovarian Syndrome) develop UFH during their teens or early 20s. PCOS is the most common hormonal disorder among women of reproductive age in the U.S.

- An estimated 70 percent of postmenopausal women who are not taking hormone replacement therapy will develop UFH, with changes in the androgen-to-estrogen ratio.

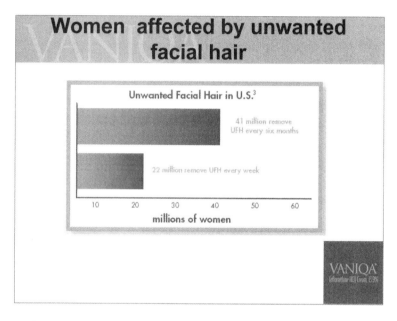

Where to Get More Information About Hirsutism

Your doctor is the best resource for finding out important information related to your particular case *(your obstetrician/gynecologist [OBGYN] is also a good resource)*. Not all patients with hirsutism are alike, and it is important that your situation is evaluated by someone who knows you as a whole person. A number of Web sites on the Internet have information about hirsutism as well. Information provided by the National Institutes of Health, National Medical Societies, and some other well-established organizations are often reliable sources of information, although the frequency with which their information is updated is variable.

◆ National Library of Medicine
www.nlm.nih.gov/med lineplus

◆ The Hormone Foundation www.hormone.org

- www.hirsutism.homestead.com
- www.bouldermedicalcenter.com/Articles/Hirsutism.htm
- www.patients.update.com

SEE CHAPTER 21 FOR MORE RESOURCES

How This Book Can Help You

This book can help you in many ways. I have gathered the information over the past 18 years. Some of the statistics are courtesy of SkinMedica Inc. and Palomar Medical Technologies, as well as reliable Internet resources. The remaining information is from my life experiences, personal interviews and years of hands-on experience working as an electrologist and certified medical laser technician.

The information in this book can help you:

- Realize that you are NOT alone.
- Understand *why* and *how* hair grows.
- Analyze your specific *condition* and the severity of it.
- Enable you to face and accept your condition.
- Get diagnosed properly, preventing further adverse side effects from a disorder that you didn't even know you had.
- Start the healing the process—from inside out!
- Understand and become educated about the many treatment options available today.
- Formulate the APPROPRIATE treatment plan tailored to your specific needs.

- Design your "realistic expectations" on becoming smoother!
- Permanently reduce unwanted hair growth.
- Save time, money and aggravation by not having to remove hair on a daily basis with tedious, temporary methods of hair removal.
- Look and feel better about yourself and your appearance.
- Attain a healthier, more productive lifestyle.

CHAPTER 1

MY PERSONAL BATTLE: LAURA'S STORIES

**"A battle sometimes decides everything; and sometimes the most trifling thing decides the fate of a battle."
—Napoleon Bonaparte**

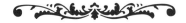

"Hurricane Hairy"

I feel it is important to get my story out to the public. It is not common to talk about this topic; therefore, the condition in general does not get the attention it deserves. Women need to seek help, especially if they have a real medical problem that is causing their condition. Maybe this book can help some women catch a possible disorder early on and prevent any further side effects, both mentally and physically.

I have some analogies that I use to try to put the level of embarrassment of being "hairy" into perspective. I would like to share these analogies with both the "hairy" and the "hairless" alike. As a young girl I was teased about my facial hair, and it was extremely painful. I hope my stories and the analogies I have included make it utterly clear just how devastating it is to be "hairy." I want to prove that the psychological effects are very real but are often disregarded or overlooked. I would like people to be able to understand the physical and emotional trauma "hairy people" feel when someone teases them or rudely points out their hair (if you are hairy, you are aware of it and you don't need someone pointing it out to you!). The first time someone says to you (especially in a public forum or social situation) something like "Wow, you have a lot of hair on your face," or "Why do you have a beard?" there is a tidal wave of embarrassment that cannot easily be defined by words. The tidal wave blows over eventually, but the damage it leaves behind is comparable to a Category 5 hurricane. The structure of how we view ourselves and the very core of who we are is completely destroyed. It can take years to rebuild some of our self-esteem, only to be hit again, and again, and again by "Hurricane Hairy".

In order to comprehend and relate to this pain, picture yourself at the most important event of your life. Pretend you are a movie star and you are about to receive your Academy

Award. You are shining on the red carpet! You are dressed in a designer gown and shoes, and the entire world has its eyes fixed on you. Flashes from countless cameras go off and people are chanting your name. It is the most amazing moment of your life! Then, out of nowhere, a fan yells out as loud as possible, "Hey! You have a huge booger hanging out of your nose!" Then, your designer dress malfunctions and one of your boobs bursts out of your dress! You try to stay calm, but as you try to casually walk away, the heel on one of your Manolo Blahnik shoes snaps! Now you start to panic. You bend over to try to fix your shoe and you accidentally break wind!

This is my "booger/boob/break-wind" emotion (BBB for short). Now take this feeling, multiply it by about 1,000, and now you have an emotion equivalent to what one would feel after hearing "Lady, why do you have a beard?" This might sound extreme, but from my own personal experiences, as well as the experiences of the dozens of women I interviewed, the level of embarrassment is so profound, and this comparison seems to capture those intense emotions. Most people can understand and relate to the embarrassing feelings associated with boogers and accidental bodily functions. This analogy is meant to accentuate the fact that being "hairy" can be significantly more embarrassing than even the most embarrassing of all situations. Now you can read my stories and truly relate to how I felt in each one.

Charlie the Chin Hair

Teenage existence is difficult enough without noticing one day that you have a hair on your face. I called the first one "Charlie"—Charlie the chin hair. It was funny—he was sort of my friend for a while. That was until Charlie became a party animal and invited his friends, family, distant relatives, and eventually the entire East Coast to hang out on my face! Charlie became a real "pain in the neck" (and chin and lip and so on) and I really started to despise him. This was a crucial and delicate point in my life. My hormones were raging, I was struggling to "fit in," and I was both physically and emotionally unstable, as many teens can be. Social acceptance and how we look is critical. I had a hard time being one of the girls because I would look in the mirror and see a boy—a big, hairy, scary beast of a boy, no less. I was the one in the group who got left out of the inner circle and was often made fun of. My so-called friends had terrible nicknames for me. I dug deep into my memory bank to remember some of these names, but I obviously managed to block these out, hoping to delete them from my memory. I buried the cutting words so deep away that I can't find them anymore. I know they were harsh; I know they hurt me; I know it is best that I don't remember them. Needless to say, they were nicknames that involved the hairs on my face (lip, chin, neck, buttocks, and even my abdomen and breasts at one point). I wouldn't change my clothes in front of my friends. ALL young girls try on clothes and "get naked" in front of each other, but not hairy scary Laura—no way!

As time passed, I began to shave, pluck, bleach and wax, and I also purchased every ridiculous infomercial concoction that promised smoothness. What I ultimately did was create a beast! I created a person so ashamed of herself that I began to retreat into an isolated, empty, hopeless world. I wouldn't go on vacations with my friends if it involved the beach or having to share a room with other girls. Of course, I used the excuse of strict parents because there was NO WAY I could share a house and one bathroom with five or six other girls AND control my facial and body hair. It would take hours to meticulously pluck and shave, only to be riddled with bleeding razor rashes and lumpy plucking marks. It was time-consuming and incredibly stressful. It was simply not physically possible. At this point I truly evolved into "Laura the Sasquatch." My femininity was compromised and I felt very masculine. Dark, coarse, dreadful hair covered my body from head to toe. I was blessed with a lot of hair on my head so I was lucky in that respect, but unfortunately, my long, thick, enviable tresses did not make me feel any less like a Sasquatch. I couldn't go to the beach with razor burn on my face, butt, bikini line and countless other places. I just couldn't do it, and I missed out on a lot of fun and parties and trips with my friends. Society and relentless teenagers were intolerant of anything outside the "norm." The beautiful models on the magazine covers only had mustaches if a bored kid decided to doodle on his mom's magazine. My generation of "Sasquatches" had no role models. NOBODY talked about face and body hair. There was (and still is) no famous "hairy" person to look up to. It was a non-existent topic, and I felt utterly alone. I missed much of the excitement of being young. I was robbed of fun and freedom and the opportunity to wear short shorts and be a happy and free teenager! You are probably feeling pretty sorry for me, right? Well, don't, because I am absolutely grateful to every single hair that ever popped out of my body. I am a better woman today because of what I went through, and now I get to take this energy and help change this taboo topic into a more commonly discussed issue. The pain and anger and seclusion gave me an inner desire to CHANGE THE WORLD (in a small sense of course).

At this point, I started doing research on methods of permanent hair removal, which led me to find Harriett (I did call her "hairy" because it was too ironic). We all have a "Harriett" in one way or another. I dedicated part of this book to her even though she probably doesn't even remember me. Harriett was an electrologist, but in my eyes, she was Wonder Woman—a real hair-fighting superhero!

Unfortunately, electrolysis treatments were expensive and it was a financial burden. In order to be able to continue electrolysis treatments on myself, I became a professional "hair remover" myself and graduated from the Berkowitz School of Electrolysis. Hair removal became my obsession. I studied hard and received my electrolysis certification and opened a small electrolysis practice in my parents' basement in Staten Island, New York. As my practice grew, I was so shocked to see just how many other women were dealing with the same problem of excessive hair growth. The obsession only grew, and I would get so much joy and satisfaction from helping other women and young girls permanently remove and reduce their deepest demon—HAIR! I watched these women evolve right in front of my eyes. Some of them would come to me on the first visit very shy and embarrassed. After a few months, I watched them blossom into happier and more confident people. It was like a miracle! I could not believe the transformation in some cases. Unfortunately, results were achieved slowly and the process was very tedious. My obsession led me to continue my education in the world of laser hair removal. The following chapters will tell the rest of the story!

Coma Phobia

I shared the following story with dozens of women, and it was astounding how many of them had a similar experience. It was so important to realize that I was not alone. I could not believe that other women felt the same exact way that I did. The story goes like this: I asked my sister (one of the very few people that were aware of my condition) to shave me should I ever become incapacitated or admitted to the hospital for any reason. I needed her to save me from the embarrassment of letting my facial and body hair (including on my legs) grow down to my feet! I didn't care if I wet the bed, soiled the sheets, vomited on myself, or even reeked of body odor, but for heaven's sake, don't let anyone see my beard because THAT would be embarrassing! Beat me, torture me, kill me—just don't let my chin hair be seen! I would never get over it, even if I were in a coma.

I suffered in silence for many years over my condition. My road to recovery has been a tough one, but has also initiated a fire in me to help find a more effective solution to this problem. The following chapters detail what I have learned over the years.

Happy "Hairy" Thanksgiving!

In order to write this chapter about my own personal stories, I had to interview my mother and ask her if she remembered anything at all about me and my "hair." I needed her to fill in the blanks of my memory because I had literally blocked out some of the more gruesome details dealing with my "hairiness." I mention this a few times throughout this book because I find it fascinating that although I can remember being hurt by situations, I can't always remember the details. Many women I interviewed also had similar cases of "selective memory."

Anyway, when I was about 16 or 17, my mom, dad, sister and I were having Thanksgiving dinner at my aunt's house. As usual, we were having fun, laughing and talking around the table as we ate dessert. While I was in the middle of biting into my delicious chocolate-covered cream puff, my male cousin, who is four years older than me, suddenly spouted out, "Ew! You have, like, a beard! What's up with that?" He was not very discreet about this. As a matter of fact, he screamed it across the table in a loud, deafening and unsympathetic voice! As my mom told me the story, I was slowly starting to remember the incident. I even clearly remember the feeling I had (similar to the "BBB" analogy?).

This was truly one of the most terrible days of my life. I secluded myself in my room for days (which felt like years), dwelling over it, crying over it, and most importantly, researching my options. Although I was anything but grateful that Thanksgiving, that day marked a turning point for me. It was the final straw that broke the "Sasquatch's" back! That was when I found Harriet the electrologist, and the rest is history! In retrospect, I am actually thankful to my cousin for "giving" me a punch in the gut, so to speak, that Thanksgiving day.

Kids Say the Darndest Things (And Then Your Life Is Ruined)

I am sure just about every human being has been embarrassed in one way or another by an overly honest child. Well, I had my share of embarrassment, as well. Once again, I had to interview someone to jog my memory. This time my husband had to tell me this story, and I think he was having a "BBB" emotion as he was slowly and ever-so-delicately telling the story. To keep it short and sweet, I was dating Andy (my husband of 10 years now) for maybe two or three months. Andy was previously married and had a son, also named Andy, who was around four years old at the time. We were still in that very impressionable period in our relationship; you know, that "Look at how wonderful I am. Don't you think I'm amazing?" stage. I knew very early on in our relationship that I would marry this man, so I was on my very "best behavior." Boy, did I do everything right! I was going to make him fall head over heels in love with me! Well, thanks to his ever-so-observant son, he fell head over heels, alright! But along the way, he tripped over my chin hair and landed on my excessively stubble-laden legs, then pulled himself up using the strings of my belly hair *(that's how I envisioned it, anyway)*.

Basically, all three of us were sitting around his kitchen table one night, just having ice cream and chatting. Then, out of nowhere, I caught this adorable little child staring at me with a confused look on his face. He slowly opened his mouth, and in a befuddled manner asked, "Why do you have a beard?"

At this point, all I need to say is close your eyes and visualize my "BBB" scenario. Get it? I bet you do. I have enabled you to physically feel exactly what I felt that day. As you read the next story, you will probably not be surprised by what occurred further down the road in our relationship……

I Love You, But…

For the grand finale, this next story is a sequel to the previous. It is by far the most devastating for me to handle. It has to do with a VERY recent secret my husband confessed to. This information is so new to me that I write each word with hesitation and a very heavy heart. When I decided to write this book, I wanted to be sure that I captured the honest emotions and psychological effects that we suffer from having excess hair growth. That meant that I had to do research and interview real people and get real stories. I began the interview process and I learned things that have sincerely changed my life. People opened up to me and trusted me; tears were shed and emotions were deep and strong. My heart went out to these people as they poured their hearts out to me and told me things that they never thought they would utter out loud. This was so overwhelming for me, and I can honestly say that I have a profoundly new outlook on life because of what Andy told me. This topic is extremely valid; this topic is even more important than I had realized; this topic is a source of implausible psychological distress and exceedingly significant self-esteem issues; this topic wound up touching my life deeper than I could have ever dreamed.

As I mentioned earlier, I interviewed my husband Andy for the book. I thought it would be interesting and even "fun." We sat down one night after the kids went off to bed. I was relaxed and comfortable in my beloved purple robe as I hunched excitedly over my laptop, eagerly awaiting his stories! I was so intrigued to finally hear his side of my "hairiness" and discuss the topic very openly and honestly. Of course, we have talked about my condition over the years, but never in a "sit down and open up" kind of way. I couldn't wait to hear what he had to say. My whole life had revolved around being hairy, and Andy had been my biggest and greatest supporter. I just had no idea that the words that would pour out of his mouth would change my whole life. I had no idea that he was holding secrets that he never shared with me. I had no idea that this man that I have known for 15 years—my husband and my best friend—had a bombshell to tell me that would shake the very core of my being.

As I type this, my fingers slip against my wet keyboard as my tears spill uncontrollably out of my eyes. I am literally shocked by these revelations. I have no analogies for this emotion! I cannot believe I am sharing this story with the world. As you know by now, I have a pretty strong self-defense mechanism for blocking out most of the deep, hurtful occurrences. The fact that I am documenting the most shocking of all my experiences and making the words real is the ultimate "closure" for me. I can finally rest at ease and move on. I know the truth to something that has tormented me for years, and ironically, it is all about my "hairiness."

I asked Andy to give me a quote or a quick story for the book—something juicy that we had never talked about before. He looked at me with the strangest look. He hesitated so I pursued him and practically forced it out of him. I continued: "Come on, I know you can come up with something good. There must be something you can tell me that would be important and relevant to the book." Well, that turned out to be quite an understatement of titanic proportions.

He hesitated again with that same look on his face. It was so obvious that what he was going to say would hurt me. He was trying so hard to be delicate. Very quietly, he told me that he was hesitant about marrying me because of my "hairiness." He admitted, after 15 years, that he actually had doubts about committing to me ONLY because of my condition. He knew he loved me very early on in our relationship. He never doubted how he felt about me as a person, but he was way more affected by the "hair" than he had ever let on. I was completely in shock. I could not believe what he was telling me.

As I soaked this in, I remembered the few occasions when Andy would pull away from our relationship and "need time alone." They were like little "mini-breakups." Out of the blue he would just tell me that he was unsure about things and that we needed to take a break. Normally, I would have quickly assumed it was the "hairiness," but I thought Andy was different. I pointed out my condition to him very early on in our relationship. Andy even drove me to my electrolysis sessions and built my office when I became an electrologist. I was sure that he was "cool" with the situation. I assumed the "mini-breakups" were because of his recently failed marriage. He was a young single father with a lot of responsibilities and went through a tough divorce. I was convinced that he was scared of committing again. I always just gave him his room and let him take time to figure out what he needed to.

We just celebrated our 10-year wedding anniversary, and we are a very strong couple. Of course, we have our challenges, but we are together for the long haul. We are truly partners in life. I can't believe I have been hit with this bombshell. How could I be so blind? How come he never told me? I am overcome with WHYs and HOWs. I feel like the past 10 years have been a lie in a way.

I wear my heart on my sleeve, so Andy was able to see my emotions and knew how shocked and devastated I was. He tried to console me, and we talked for hours. He explained that he loved me as a person and how that always outweighed any kind of "cosmetic" issues. He said he also knew deep down that he was going to spend the rest of his life with me, but he took those "mini-breakups" to just sort it out within himself and come to terms with the fact that I was "hairy." He told me that the hair on my face was not even the main issue. I did so much to hide it and cover it up that it was not even noticeable most of the time. He also knew I was taking steps to permanently get rid of the facial hair with the electrolysis. Unfortunately, I was so focused on the facial hair that I guess I started to slack off on the other areas. Daily methods of hair removal were so time-consuming, and I just didn't have the energy to put into all the other areas. I guess I started to "take advantage" of the fact that I thought he accepted it. I got comfortable and wasn't as diligent in shaving my legs, bikini area, stomach and buttocks. I thought it was no big deal to him, but I was wrong, and apparently, it bothered him a great deal. He said that he would try to give me hints without being too blunt. He certainly knew that it was a sensitive and sore subject, so he did not want to blatantly hurt me.

The bottom line here is that UFH, UBH, hirsutism, and just plain "hairiness" in general are a MAJOR issue to everyone involved. Andy's story led me to wonder how many other women have actually lost "true love" because of hairiness. I was lucky, but are other hirsute women out there alone because of this? I believe the answer is a big YES, and we need to do something about it. I don't know what I would have done if I lost Andy over this. We have to give this topic attention in order to avoid further devastation.

I could write another whole book just about how this story made me feel, but I will deal with it and move on. I will get through this as I always have in the past. Just keep in mind: If you are a possible "Andy" or "Laura," it is time to seek help and do something about it! This book was written for that purpose, so use the tools wisely.

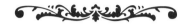

CHAPTER 2

THE HAIRS THAT BOND US: REAL PEOPLE—REAL STORIES

"Every great man is unique."
—Ralph Waldo Emerson

Take a journey with me through the lives of some of the most incredible, strong and superior women that I have met over the past 18 years. I opened my medical spa, Divine Laser Hair Removal Inc., in 2004. I am a certified electrologist and a certified medical laser technician. I have worked tirelessly since I was a young girl to find an effective, permanent solution for excessive hair growth. I have been professionally removing and reducing hair for over 15 years. I have kept journals throughout the years of my experiences and interviews with patients, family members and friends.

I am always touched by the comments I receive. To realize that these women were going through so much, and at the end of it all—after years and years of torment, treatments, hormone therapies and even surgeries in some cases—they could not consider themselves truly feminine because of the hair that still grew on their faces and bodies. Hormone therapy works wonders on slowing down the production of new hair follicles, but the follicles that already exist will remain during and after therapy is completed. So even if these women are essentially healthier and their disorders are under control, the fact that they still struggle with unwanted, excessive hair continues to deeply affect them in a negative manner. This scenario is magnified for transgender patients (see Chapter 12). On a positive note, this book will prove that there is *hope*. There are methods of permanently reducing unwanted hair, and it is the end result that gives these hirsute patients closure.

Here are just a few quotes and stories from my friends, family members and patients over the past 18 years. These women are my valiant inspirations.

❖ Anonymous, Age 38, Body Hair (Nipples, Abdomen)

"When I got out of an 11-year relationship, I wanted to do

something to make me feel younger and sexier; some extra confidence to get back into the dating game. I have always been self-conscious of the hair on my happy trail (stomach) and nipples, so that was the first thing I wanted to change to have sexier, smoother skin. Laser treatments are easy and well worth every penny. Now, for the rest of my life, I don't have to worry about unwanted hair growth in embarrassing areas."

❖ Dee, Age 60, Facial Hair and Excessive Body Hair

"My children always made fun of me for wearing old-fashioned, high-necked shirts and turtlenecks. I didn't admit it to them until recently that it was because of the hair on my chest and neck that I was afraid of showing. I was desperately fearful that people would see the hair. I felt like a beast or animal of some kind. I certainly did not feel feminine. I tried waxing, tweezing, and even electrolysis, but the hair would keep coming back. In my 40s, I was diagnosed with overactive thyroid. My doctor told me one of the side effects is facial and body hair growth, but there was nothing I could do about it. I believed him and just shaved it every day and did my best to hide it and cover it with scarves and high-necked shirts. Now that I have completed my laser treatments, I look back and can't believe how I used to feel. It is overwhelming. I felt like a monster and now I feel so open and free. I only wish I had done this years ago, but at least it is done now and I can hold my head up and wear low-cut shirts! Of course, now I have the wrinkles to cover up, but at least there is no hair growing out of them! My life has changed dramatically and I feel like I have a new face."

❖ Ann, Age 45, Facial Hair

"I never looked people in the face. I would either have my head down or my hand on my chin and neck. I had what I called a beard—literally. It started in my teens and it was a very difficult thing for me to deal with. I was tormented by it. I remember envying my friends that were blond and hairless. I was even jealous; I couldn't enjoy normal things like other girls. For instance, I was never able to just go away for a weekend on the spur of the moment. I always had to make sure I was shaved from head to toe and that I had the proper utensils, like tweezers, packed. It was exhausting keeping up with it. I thought I would never meet a man because of it."

❖ Anonymous, Age 20, Body Hair (Lower Back, Abdomen)

"I am so embarrassed by the hair on my back (lower back) and belly. I am so afraid that people will see it and make fun of me—it is one of my biggest fears."

❖ Anonymous, Age 62, Facial Hair and Excessive Body Hair

"I have been married for over 40 years. My husband has been dealing with my hirsutism practically since the day we met. He, of all people, knows what a tender topic this always was for me. Many years ago, way before I got my laser treatments, we got into a fight. We were going through a tough time and he got very mad at me one day. During an argument, he called me a name that I will never forget. He still feels bad about it, even after all these years. Those words cut me like a knife. He called me a hairy bitch; it was one of the worst days of my life. He is not a mean person, and I know he said it out of anger, but it was so hurtful. It really opened my eyes to the fact that the hair was a problem for him—I never knew that he was aware of it. I thought I hid it so well from him; until that day, he never mentioned a word about it. I don't even remember what the fight was about, but I do remember that it caused me to do something about my hair problem. About six months after this argument, we were driving in the car on a sunny day. Normally I would be horrified to be in the bright light because it would enhance the hairs on my face, but I just got my third laser treatment and I was so much smoother. My husband looked over at me and told me I looked extra beautiful and asked me if I had done something different to my hair or something like that. He couldn't quite place what was different about me, but he sure noticed something. I think I was just glowing and more confident and not holding my head down. I felt redeemed. That was one of the better days of my life. When I look back now, I am actually glad he called me that name because it gave me such a determination to get rid of the hair. I had no idea how much different I would feel about myself."

CHAPTER 3

UNDERSTANDING THE ENEMY: ANATOMY OF A HAIR FOLLICLE

"Most people spend more time and energy in going around problems than in trying to solve them."
—Henry Ford

If you are finally ready to do something about excessive hair growth, I highly recommend learning the nitty-gritty details of WHY you have the hair growth and HOW it got there. Once you understand the WHYs and HOWs, the treatment options and expectations make more sense. You should be armed with knowledge in order to properly treat your condition. This book is intended to educate you and arm you with the ammunition you need to combat your condition and walk away victorious! It is very easy to ignore something when you simply don't understand it. I tried so many treatments that promised permanent results throughout my teens and early twenties, only to fail each time. I truly believe it was the lack of knowledge that caused the failures. You must know WHY you have a problem. It can determine the type of treatment plan that you should obtain. You should know HOW hair grows so you can get treatments at the proper intervals which will help you get real results as well as save you time and money.

Have you ever wondered why there is no simple cure for hirsutism? Have you ever sat in front of your mirror (your big 20x magnification mirror), tediously plucking those hairs and thinking, *Why can't we find a cure for this?* After all, we can do miraculous things like walk on the moon and genetically clone another human being, but we can't stop hair from growing! Hair growth seems so simple, right? It seems silly that we don't have a cure for it! Why can't we just invent a pill or cream to stop it overnight? Well, that is the misconception. Hair growth is not simple. The entire process is extremely complicated and clinically tedious. You will definitely achieve better results once you are educated on this very complicated process. Unfortunately, there is not an abundance of readily available resources on the topic. As a matter of fact, I personally feel that the entire topic of unwanted and excessive hair is terribly neglected. Once we start to OPENLY talk about it and admit to it, we can give it the attention it deserves. Here is a condensed version of "Hair Growth 101" (courtesy of Skin Medica)

Anatomy of a Hair Follicle

Hair follicles develop when epithelial cells grow (downward) into the dermis/subcutis from the epidermis. The deepest part of the epithelial downgrowth becomes the germination point of hair growth, termed the germinal matrix. The germinal matrix grows over and around a papilla of the dermal connective tissue, creating an anatomical "ball and socket" type of arrangement. The dermal papilla is rich in capillaries which nourish the germinal matrix. The germinal matrix (socket) and dermal papilla (ball) together are referred to as the follicular bulb. The part of the epidermal downgrowth that connects the germinal matrix with the skin surface forms a canal and is called the external root sheath. Hair growth is accomplished by the growth of the germinal matrix epithelia cells, which push upward toward the skin surface through the canal. As the germinal cells push upwards, the outermost layer of the hair, composed of soft keratin, becomes the internal root sheath. This sheath only extends partway up the follicle.

The portion of a hair extending outside the skin is called the hair shaft. The part of the hair embedded in the skin is the hair root. Sebaceous glands are present in the upper dermis surrounding the follicle and secrete sebum into the follicular canal to lubricate the hair. The hairs of all but the beard and pubic regions have an associated bundle of smooth muscle referred to as the arrector pili muscle (erector of hair). Contraction of this muscle causes "goose bumps" and also

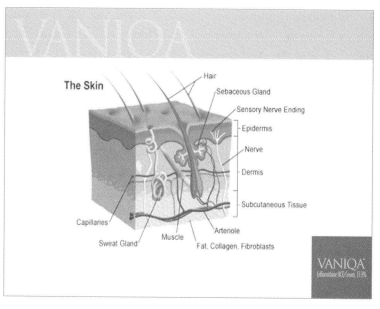

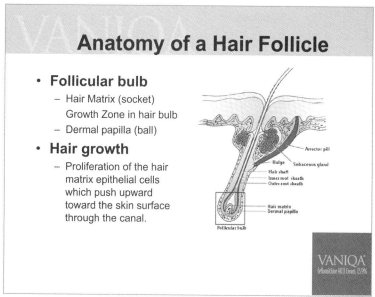

squeezes the sebaceous gland, which lies between the arrector pili and the follicle, initiating the secretion of sebum.

The major component of hair is a protein known as keratin. The hair shaft is made up of thin fibers of keratin twisted together into thicker bundles. A transverse section of hair reveals that hair is made up of three distinct layers. The innermost layer is the medulla, the middle layer is the cortex, and the outermost layer is the cuticle.

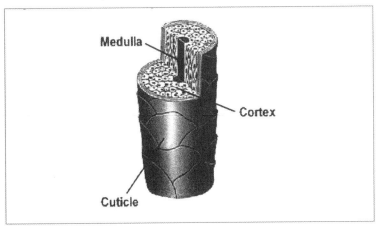

- Medulla: thin layer in the center of the hair. Not always present the entire length of the hair shaft.
- Cortex: middle layer comprising the bulk of the hair shaft. Composed of keratinizing epithelial cells bound together.
- Cuticle: the outermost, thin layer of overlapping epithelial cells. Relatively impermeable.

Life Cycle of Hair

Hair follicles undergo through three phases of hair growth: anagen, catagen and telogen.

Anagen is the *growth* phase of the follicle cycle. During anagen, chemical signals from the dermal papilla attract keratinocytes to grow downward through the dermis to the level of subcutis (hypodermis), forming the germinal matrix. The enzyme, ornithine decarboxylase (ODC), *present only during anagen*, causes the matrix keratinocytes to divide and produce hard keratin, forming hair. The anagen phase of hair growth is the phase most susceptible to chemical intervention. Anagen can last from several months to years.

> **KEYPOINT: Follicles can only be permanently destroyed (killed) during the anagen phase. Only a percentage of hairs are in the anagen phase at any given time—this is why NUMEROUS treatments of any form of permanent hair removal or reduction are required.**

Catagen is a relatively brief, transitional phase of hair growth, lasting from about two to four weeks. During catagen, the hair growth *slows and stops*. Lack of ODC results in cessation of keratinocyte cell division and, eventually, atrophy (decrease) of the germinal matrix. The hair root detaches from the germinal matrix and the hair begins to undergo expulsion from the follicle.

Telogen is referred to as the resting phase of hair growth. Telogen lasts from three to six months; *no hair growth* takes place during this phase. All cellular mechanisms of hair growth are inactive during telogen. By the end of telogen, the hair is loosely attached to the follicle and can usually be easily pulled out by brushing or washing the hair. Chemical compounds do not have an effect during telogen.

> **KEYPOINT: These phases make it difficult to know the true total amount of hair that you really have. Only a percentage of the hair that you have is above the skin and visible to you at any given time. This is misleading because you actually have more hair than you think you have.**

Hair Growth Cycle

- Anagen: **Growing Phase**
  - Can last several months to years
  - Most susceptible to chemical compounds
  - The enzyme ODC is present
- Catagen:**Transitional Phase**
  - Last several weeks
  - Hair growth slows and stops
- Telogen: **Resting Phase**
  - Lasts several months
  - No hair growth takes place
  - Chemical compounds do not have an effect

The life span of hair varies. Hair follicles of the scalp have a longer cycle than those of the face. For example, scalp hair anagen lasts from 2 to 6 years, while lip hair anagen lasts from 4 to 14 weeks. The transitional phase (catagen) and resting phase (telogen) of lip and scalp are similar, with catagen lasting up to two weeks and telogen lasting from one to three months. Hairs on different parts of the body are "programmed" specifically for their body location. In fact, it has been shown that transplanted hairs retain their original life cycle program.

> **KEYPOINT: Because of these variations, the process of permanently removing and reducing hair is made increasingly difficult. Each individual person has their own cycle durations which further complicate treatment timing.**

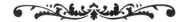

CHAPTER 4

WHY AM I SO HAIRY?

"A good scare is worth more to a man than good advice."
—E.E. Howe

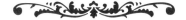

Why am I so hairy? I have asked myself this question hundreds of times since I was a tender, "fuzzy" 15-year-old girl. I am now 36 years old and have been through many turning points in my life. The answer to this question has evolved and even morphed over the years. Some of the more memorable and even borderline *insane* answers have been:

- Because.
- It is from my Italian heritage.
- I deserve it.
- I have no idea.
- Hairy women are "sexy."
- I am cursed.
- I use it as protection from being promiscuous.
- It is my mother's fault.
- I started shaving and waxing, which caused more hair to grow.
- I am not normal.

The list is actually longer, but can also be quite boring! It turns out that these ridiculous answers were way out of line and far from reality. The point here is that there truly was a valid, clinical answer to the mentally and physically debilitating question of "Why Am I So Hairy?" The answers that I concocted were just excuses that I used to avoid the real truth. The truth was something that I was utterly afraid to deal with. The answer was so important, yet I was so overshadowed by despair, embarrassment and denial that I was completely blind to it.

KEYPOINT: We have to educate and make women and young girls AWARE that avoiding and covering up UFH and UBH can be harmful.

The "answer" for me was a medical disorder called PCOS *(Polycystic Ovarian Syndrome).* This diagnosis was profoundly important to my mental and physical health, but it took me years to figure it out because of my lack of awareness and education. We will learn more about the different disorders that cause hirsutism and their definitions as we proceed. Please stick with me; I will expose you to topics, issues, symptoms, real stories, diagnosis and, ultimately, the attainable treatment options and viable solutions that you have been searching for!

"Scared Smooth"

I used to just say that I was "hairy," but I had no idea what that really meant from a clinical standpoint. In order to start to "de-hair" yourself and seriously begin to get some results, you should become more familiar with some of the more clinical terms for "being hairy." In my case, I started taking my condition much more seriously once I learned that my "hairiness" had a real medical name. It helped me put the severity of my condition into perspective. It truly made the difference for me. For example, when I was just "hairy," I simply "removed the hair." Once I understood that I suffered from a condition called *hirsutism* due to a disorder called *PCOS,* I got scared and seriously wanted to address my condition and treat my disorder. This new term—*hirsutism*—made me get serious! It was a great push in the right direction. *Hirsutism* and *Polycystic Ovarian Syndrome* allowed me to focus my energy into **permanently reducing** my *hirsutism* instead of covering it up, avoiding it and temporarily removing it.

At present, I have permanently destroyed a very large number of hair follicles to the point that I no longer shave or tweeze most parts of my body, including my face, underarms, happy trail (abdomen), bikini line and legs. I am triumphant and I am smooth, and I owe it all to being scared to death of remaining *hirsute* (instead of just hairy)! I guess you can say I was "scared smooth"!

Clinical Names, Official Terms and Definitions for Excessive Hair Growth:

Familiarize yourself with some of the more common and official clinical terms for "being hairy":

• **Androgenic Hair**—The hair follicles on much of the body respond to androgens (primarily testosterone and its derivatives). The rate of hair growth increases and the heaviness of the hairs increases. However, different areas respond with different sensitivities. As puberty progresses, the sequence of appearance of sexual (androgenic) hair reflects the gradations of androgen sensitivity. The pubic area is most sensitive, and heavier hair usually grows there first in response to androgens. The following regions also respond to androgens, in order of decreasing sensitivity: axillary (armpit) and perianal areas, sideburns, above the upper lip, periareolar areas, chin and beard areas, center of the chest, arms and legs, across the chest, shoulders, buttocks, back, and abdomen.

• **UFH**—Unwanted Facial Hair

• **UBH**—Unwanted Body Hair

• **Hirsutism** (pronounced hur-suh-tih-zum) is often characterized by "male-patterned" body hair, though it is extremely common in females. It is excessive hair growth of terminal hair (long, coarse hair) in androgen-dependent areas of a woman's body where terminal hair is not normally found, including the face, neck, chest, lower abdomen, back, upper arms, upper legs and inner thighs. Elevated androgen levels (testosterone and dihydrotestosterone) result in increased vellus and terminal hair growth, as well as increased conversion of vellus to terminal hair. Hirsutism is a chronic condition, most commonly hereditary or familial (See Chapter 6 for causes of hirsutism).

• **Idiopathic or Famialial Hirsutism** involves a distribution of hair growth which is not typically androgenic. Similarly, non-androgen-dependant hair growth occurs with drugs such as phenytoin, diazoxide, minoxidil and cyclosporin. **Iatrogenic Hirsutism** also occurs after treatment with androgens or more weakly androgenic drugs such as progestagens or danazol. The diagnosis of Idiopathic Hirsutism is given to women with hirsutism and no other clinical abnormalities. The serum androgen concentrations in these women are more often within the normal range than are the concentrations in women with definable causes of hirsutism.

> **KEYPOINT: *Idiopathic Hirsutism and PCOS are the major causes of hirsutism. Idiopathic Hirsutism is found in 5 to 15 percent of hirsute patients. Neither is a life-threatening disorder. However, they are not usually reversible, and the cumulative effect of chronic androgen excess typically causes a gradual increase in hair growth with age if untreated.**

• **Hypertrichosis** (pronounced hi-per-trick-o-sis) is excess hair growth, typically in non-androgen-dependent areas; the ear lobe, for example. Hypertrichosis can be inherited. Late-onset hypertrichosis is commonly associated with medication side effects. A diagnosis of hypertrichosis may be used on hair growth pattern, lack of elevated circulating androgens, and familial history.

• **Localized Hypertrichosis**—In some cases, an area of skin can react to repeated trauma or to some other asymmetric stimulus (such as wearing of a cast) with increased hair growth.

- **Virulism**—When hirsutism is associated with recession of the hairline, deepening of the voice, loss of female body shape, and the development of male-pattern pubic hair, it is called **virulism.**

Why Our Body Actually "Needs" Hair: Normal Hair Pattern and Growth

There are two types of hair on the body: (1) vellus hairs which are short, fine and colorless, and (2) terminal hairs which are long, coarse, colored and, in certain areas of the body, responsive to hormonal influence (androgens).

The adrenal gland and the ovary normally make androgens (male hormones). In normal amounts, androgens cause acne and the appearance of terminal hair on the extremities, armpits and pubic area at the time of puberty.

It is important to remember that all human beings are "supposed" to have hair for the purpose of protection. Nearly all the skin of the human body, except the palms of the hands and the soles of the feet, are covered with hairs *(usually Vellus hairs).* The density of the hairs (in hair follicles per square centimeter), thickness, color, speed of growth and quality of the hair, such as kinkiness, vary from one part of the body to another and from one person to another. All of these features have strong genetic determinants, as demonstrated by the inheritability of these qualities.

> **KEYPOINT: You will always have some form of hair growth on your body. Completing a full treatment plan of electrolysis, laser or IPL treatments will probably greatly reduce the darker hairs, but the treated areas may still have the lighter vellus hairs.**

At birth, we all have a predetermined number of hair follicles. Not all follicles are in an active stage (anagen) at one time (many can remain dormant for a long time). This is very important to know because it can help you set your realistic expectations (Chapter 14), understand the progress of your treatments, and ultimately, be satisfied with the **LONG-TERM RESULTS**.

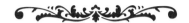

CHAPTER 5

SYMPTOMS, EVALUATION AND DIAGNOSIS

"Is is part of the cure to want to be cured."
—Seneca

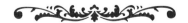

You must accept the fact that you are "hairy." Owning up to "your hairiness" will equip you with the confidence you need to vocalize your desire to get rid of the hair and seek professional help. You will be able to push aside your embarrassment and TALK TO YOUR DOCTOR. Start with your family doctor or OBGYN if you prefer. They may be able to diagnose you properly or refer you to the proper specialist. If you truly have a disorder, you must seek help from an endocrinologist (or a pediatric endocrinologist for children) for further evaluation and treatment.

Symptoms

A woman with the mildest form of hirsutism may notice significant growth of hair that is mature (the same color as scalp hair) on the upper lip, chin, sideburn area, around the nipples or on the lower abdomen. More advanced hirsutism will cause mature hair to grow on the upper back, shoulders, sternum and upper abdomen. It most often begins during puberty. If hirsutism starts before or after puberty, the cause could be hormonal and the woman should be evaluated by a doctor.

There are many disorders that can cause hirsutism; therefore, there are many symptoms. Here is a breakdown of symptoms by disorder:

- Polycystic Ovarian Syndrome (PCOS)—Women with PCOS often have hirsutism in combination with acne, balding near the front of their head, and menstrual irregularities. PCOS is also associated with other medical problems, such as infertility due to the irregular menstrual cycles, obesity, diabetes mellitus, high cholesterol levels, and possibly heart disease. It is important to identify any or all of these problems, because effective treatments are available.
- Idiopathic Hirsutism—Idiopathic Hirsutism refers

to hirsutism that has no identifiable cause. Doctors suspect that it may be a mild variation of PCOS, and like PCOS, idiopathic hirsutism is usually chronic. A gradual, increased growth of coarse body hair is typically the only symptom in women with this condition. Menstrual cycles are always normal in women with idiopathic hirsutism.

For disorders other than PCOS, some of the more common symptoms that accompany excessive hair growth can include one or more of the following:

- If a woman's androgen level is very high, she may experience male pattern balding, decreased breast size, and a deepening of her voice.

- Most patients with hirsutism will have some disturbance of menstruation (like missed periods). The greater the disruption, the more likely it is that there is a serious cause.

- Many patients with hirsutism are also overweight or obese. This worsens the underlying androgen excess and insulin resistance and inhibits the response to treatment, and is an indication for appropriate advice on diet and exercise. In severe cases, the insulin resistance may have a visible manifestation as acanthosis nigricans on the neck and in the axillae.

- Other less common signs/symptoms may include: –Hair thinning (on the top of the head) –Skin tags under the armpits or neck area –High total cholesterol and/or low HDL "good cholesterol" –High blood pressure –Pre-diabetes, or in some cases, diabetes

Evaluation and Diagnosis

> **KEYPOINT: If you suffer from hirsutism AND have one or more symptoms mentioned above, it is important to see your doctor for an evaluation. Remember, you are your bodies best representative. Don't let it down! If you think something is wrong with you- voicalize it. This book will give you symptoms, diagnosis' as well as tests that you must take in order to get diagnosed. Speak-up and ask your doctor for specific tests if he is not offering them!**

The doctor will ask you about your medical history with special attention to your menstrual cycles. He or she also will examine you. If you have a normal cyclic pattern of menstrual periods, the hirsutism is most likely genetic (inherited). If your menstrual cycles are irregular and have always been irregular, the cause could be polycystic ovarian syndrome. If the hirsutism and menstrual irregularity are new, you will need to be evaluated for a potentially more serious condition, such as a tumor of the ovary, adrenal glands or pituitary gland. This is especially important if you are skipping periods. If you have mild hirsutism and don't have any symptoms that suggest you are significantly overproducing androgen hormones, you may not need any additional testing. Often, this is enough to establish a diagnosis. The diagnosis is confirmed with further laboratory testing and possible radiological studies.

Traditionally, patients with hirsutism have been divided into those with no elevation of serum androgen levels and no other clinical features (usually labeled "idiopathic hirsutism"), and those with an identifiable endocrine imbalance (most commonly polycystic ovarian syndrome, PCOS, or rarely other causes). However, in recent years it has become apparent upon more detailed investigation that most patients with "idiopathic hirsutism" have some radiological or biochemical evidence of PCOS.

A variety of investigations may aid the diagnosis of patients with hirsutism. You are likely to have several blood tests to look for the following:

- The hormones testosterone and dehydroepiandrosterone may be measured to check for signs of polycystic ovarian syndrome, ovarian tumors, adrenal gland tumors, adrenal gland hormone deficiencies (causing overgrowth, or hyperplasia, of the adrenal glands), or tumors that can stimulate the adrenal glands. Serum DHEA-S determinations are used as a marker of adrenal androgen output, since serum concentrations vary less than do DHEA-S levels with diurnal serum cortisol levels. Moderate elevations suggest an adrenal origin for the hirsutism.

- The hormone prolactin may be measured to check for signs of a tumor in the pituitary gland.

- Blood sugar and cholesterol levels may be tested, because diabetes and high levels of cholesterol commonly are associated with some causes of hirsutism.

- Gonadotrophin levels. LH hypersecretion is a consistent feature of PCOS, but the pulsatile nature of secretion of this hormone means that an increased LH/FSH ratio is not always observed on a random sample.

- Oestrogen levels. Oestradiol is usually normal in PCOS, but oestrone levels (which are rarely measured) are elevated due to peripheral conversion. Levels are variable in other causes.

- Test for luteinizing hormone (LH) and follicle-stimulating hormone (FSH).

- Often, in women with PCOS, luteinizing hormone (LH) levels are elevated and follicle-stimulating hormone (FSH) levels are depressed, which results in elevated LH/FSH ratios (>2 is common).

- Women with late-onset CAH usually have a normal LH/FSH ratio.

- A 17-hydroxyprogesterone level greater than 800 ng/dL is diagnostic for 21-hydroxylase deficiency, the most common defect associated with late-onset CAH.

- An intermediate 17-hydroxyprogesterone level (200-800 ng/dL per distribution of lesions) requires a dexamethasone suppression test.

- If a patient is oligomenorrheic (abnormal menstruation), LH, FSH, prolactin, and thyroid-stimulating hormone levels may be useful in the diagnosis.

- Perform a 24-hour urinary cortisol or an overnight dexamethasone suppression test if Cushing's syndrome is suggested.

- Other androgens. Androstenedione and DHEA sulphate are frequently elevated in PCOS, and even more elevated in congenital adrenal hyperplasia and virilizing tumors.

Depending on the results of these tests, your doctor may order additional hormone tests for evaluating the function of your adrenal gland and pituitary gland in order to help clarify the reason you are producing too much androgen. In some cases, your doctor will want to see a picture of one or more organs. Commonly used tests include magnetic resonance imaging (MRI) of the brain, a computed tomography (CT) scan of the adrenal glands, or an ultrasound of the ovaries.

> **KEYPOINT: If PCOS is suspected, the most consistent investigation is an ovarian ultrasound. The typical ultrasonic features are those of a thickened capsule, multiple 3-5mm cysts and hyperechogenic stroma. It should also be noted that prolonged hyperandrogenization from any cause may lead to polycystic changes in the ovary. Ultrasound may also reveal virilization ovarian tumors, although these are often small.**

*If a virilization tumour is suspected clinically or after investigation, then more complex tests may include dexamethosone suppression tests, CT or MRI or adrenals, and selective venous-sampling catheters.

Differential Diagnosis

In summary, most patients exhibiting a combination of hirsutism and menstrual disturbances will be shown to have polycystic ovarian syndrome, but the rarer alternative diagnoses should always be kept in mind and excluded with appropriate investigations if suspected. This includes late-onset CAH (early-onset, raised serum 17-x-OH-progesterone), Cushing's syndrome (look for other clinical features) and virilization tumors of the ovaries or adrenals.

The extent of investigation will depend on clinical context. In many cases a single serum testosterone may be sufficient to exclude rare causes. Urine-free cortisol should be measured if Cushing's syndrome is a clinical possibility.

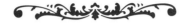

CHAPTER 6

CAUSES AND DISORDERS
(and even MORE Symptoms!)

"Some griefs are medicinal."
—William Shakespeare

Pathophysiology (The scientific study of functional changes)

Some of the following material is repetitive but I feel it is necessary to go over certain issues a few times. As you have learned, Hirsutism can be caused by abnormally high androgen levels or by hair follicles that are more sensitive than usual to normal androgen levels. Therefore, increased hair growth often is observed in patients with endocrine disorders characterized by *hyperandrogenism*. The disorders may be caused by abnormalities of the ovaries or adrenal glands. Serum levels of free testosterone, the biologically active androgen that causes hair growth, are regulated by sex hormone–binding globulin (SHBG). Lower levels of SHBG increase the availability of free testosterone. SHBG levels decrease in response to the following:

- Exogenous androgens.
- Certain disorders affect androgen levels (such as PCOS—polycystic ovarian syndrome).
- Congenital or delayed-onset adrenal hyperplasia.
- Cushing's syndrome.
- Obesity.
- Hyperinsulinemia.
- Hyperprolactinemia.
- Excess growth hormone.
- Hypothyroidism.

See definitions for these disorders below.

Conversely, SHBG levels increase with higher estrogen levels, such as the levels that occur during oral contraceptive therapy. The resultant increased SHBG levels lower the activity of circulating testosterone.

53

The severity of hirsutism does not correlate with the level of increased circulating androgens because of individual differences in androgen sensitivity of the hair follicle.

Androgen Activity

Testosterone stimulates hair growth, increasing size and intensifying the pigmentation of hair. Estrogens act in opposition, slowing growth and producing finer lighter hairs. Progesterone has minimal effect on hair growth.

The physiologic mechanism proposed for androgenic activity consists of 3 stages including: (1) production of androgens by the adrenals and ovaries, (2) androgen transport in the blood on carrier proteins (principally SHBG), and (3) intracellular modification and binding to the androgen receptor.

> **KEYPOINT: When the body produces excess levels of certain hormones (testosterone, androgen and cortisol, to name a few), only ONE of the side effects is UFH and UBH. In many cases, the excess hormone production causes many other medical issues (with some being quite serious). If you suffer from hirsutism, there is a very good chance that there is something significantly "wrong" internally, and professional medical help is imperative. Consider your "hairiness" to be a warning sign that something else might be going on. Getting the proper diagnosis and treatment can help you feel even better than you had anticipated!**

In short, central overproduction of androgen, increased peripheral conversion of androgen, decreased metabolism, and enhanced receptor binding each are potential causes of hirsutism. For circulating testosterone to exert its stimulatory effects on the hair follicle, it first must be converted into its more potent follicle-active metabolite, dihydrotestosterone.

The enzyme 5-alpha-reductase, which is found in the hair follicle, performs this conversion.

IN SUMMARY: Excessive, unwanted hair growth is caused by the production of excess levels of certain hormones, or if hair follicles are extra-sensitive to androgen.

This is the "cause." There are many disorders that cause the "cause." Here is a breakdown of some of the disorders (***PLEASE NOTE: The disorders below are some of the more common, but there may be other disorders not mentioned. Every situation is unique, so please be sure to consult with your physician to be properly diagnosed*):**

- **Congenital Adrenal Hyperlasia (CAH)**—The most "adrenal" cause of unwanted hair. CAH is a group of inherited disorders involving abnormal production of the steroid hormones— cortisol, aldosterone and androgen—by the adrenal glands. These disorders are due to a defect in one or more of the enzymes needed to make these hormones. CAH is inherited in an autosomal recessive manner. This means that a child must inherit one defective gene from each parent in order to develop the disease. CAH is a chronic condition and is usually treated with corticosteroids.

- **Cornelia de Lange Syndrome (CDLS)**—CDLS is a rare genetic disorder that leads to severe developmental anomalies. It is known to affect both physical and intellectual development in a child. The exact cause of the disease is yet to be diagnosed— but to the best of medical prognosis so far, it is termed to be a genetic disorder that most probably arises out of a faulty gene known as chromosome 3. CDLS is a congenital syndrome, meaning it is present from birth. Most of the signs and symptoms may be recognized at birth or shortly thereafter. A child need not demonstrate each and every sign or symptom for the diagnosis to be made.

As with other syndromes, individuals with CDLS strongly resemble one another. Common characteristics include: low birth weight (often under five pounds), slow growth and small stature, and small head size (microcephaly). Typical facial features include thin eyebrows which frequently meet at midline (synophrys), long eyelashes, short upturned nose, and thin, down-turned lips.

Other frequent findings include excessive body hair (hirsutism), small hands and feet, partial joining of the second and third toes, incurved fifth fingers, gastroesophageal reflux, seizures, heart defects, cleft palate, bowel abnormalities, feeding difficulties, and developmental delay. Limb differences—including missing limbs or portions of limbs (usually fingers, hands or forearms)—are also found in some individuals.

- **Congenital Generalized Hypertrichosis (CGH or Werewolf Syndrome)**—CGH is an extremely rare disorder characterized by excessive hair growth on the face and upper body, for which reason it has been dubbed "werewolf syndrome" by the popular press. Individuals with this rare phenotype have in the past appeared in circuses as "dog men" and "ape men."

- **Crash Dieting**—Women who crash diet (especially young women) can throw off their hormone balance to the point where ovulation ceases and testosterone production is increased. These women, too, may sprout a fuzzy upper lip or coarse hair elsewhere on their bodies.

- **Cushing's Disease (Cushing's Syndrome)**—Excess cortisol (an adrenal hormone) production can cause hirsutism, obesity, high blood pressure, easy bruising, and purple stretch marks.

- **Ethnicity/Race**—When it comes to the amount of body hair, there is a wide range of "normal" among women. Race and ethnicity play a major role in the growth of body hair: For example, Asian and Native American women tend to have little body hair, whereas Middle Eastern and Mediterranean women tend to have moderate to large amounts of body hair. *This is not always 100 percent true, but it is a standard that is used.*

- **Heredity/Genetics**—Unwanted hair growth can also be a result of elevated levels of testosterone or increased sensitivity of the hair follicles to normal androgen levels. Increased sensitivity, as well as some of the disorders that cause hirsutism, can be hereditary (therefore, we associate being hairy as being hereditary, but it is usually the underlying disorder that is handed down).

- **Hyperandrogenic-Insulin Resistant-Acanthosis Nigricans (hairian) Syndrome**—An endocrine condition in women that causes excessive androgen secretion. Other than excessive hair growth, symptoms can be darkening skin around the neck and underarms.

- **Hyperandrogenism**—The increased production of androgen (male type) hormones in women. However, sometimes hyperandrogenism can also involve a decrease in androgen hormone antagonists such as sex hormone-binding globulin (SHBG).

- **Hyperinsulinemia**—An endocrine disorder characterized by a failure of our Blood Sugar Control

System (BSCS) to work properly. It manifests when insulin progressively loses its effectiveness in sweeping the blood glucose from the blood stream into the 67 trillion or so cells that constitute our bodies. This means you have too much insulin in your blood. It isn't diabetes. But hyperinsulinemia is often associated with type 2 diabetes.

- **Hyperprolactinemia**—A condition of elevated serum prolactin.
- **Hyperthecosis**—An ovarian condition which is like an extreme form of PCOS. Most women with ovarian hyperthecosis are obese and have a long-standing history of hirsutism that is usually severe. Unlike PCOS, which occurs only during the reproductive years, hyperthecosis of the ovaries can occur in postmenopausal women. Hyperthecosis is often treated with anti-androgen medications. Surgery to remove the ovaries may be recommended, too, because of the associated risk of ovarian cancer.
- **Hyperthyroidism (Thyroid Conditions)**—If you suffer from an overactive thyroid gland, you have hyperthyroidism; this may increase the potency of circulating androgens, causing hirsutism. Symptoms include hair becoming rough, course, dry, breaking, brittle or falling out. Skin becomes rough, coarse, dry, scaly, itchy and thick. Puffiness and swelling around the eyes, eyelids, face, hands and feet.
- **Medications/Drugs**—Certain drugs can cause excess androgen secretion and hirsutism. If you take medications on a consistent basis, ask your doctor or pharmacist about the side effects. Some of the more common drugs that may cause hair growth include:

- ◆ Dilantin (used to control seizures).
- ◆ Danazol (used in extreme cases of endometriosis).
- ◆ Cyclosporine.
- ◆ Steroids (used in a variety of drugs, particularly asthma medications).
- ◆ Oral contraceptives (certain oral contraceptives can increase circulating androgen levels, while others decrease them).

- **Menopause**—(I pronounce this as MEAN—O—PAUSE).

  Menopause is the medical term for the end of a woman's menstrual periods. It is a natural part of aging. Low estrogen levels are linked to some uncomfortable symptoms in many women. Along with the hot flashes, mood changes and irregular periods, many women also notice changes in their skin and hair during menopause. Increased growth of hair on the face of women just before and just after menopause is quite a common occurrence. Again, these symptoms are primarily because of decreased estrogens. Below is information regarding the "normal" amounts of horones women should have. (Information from healthatoz.com):

KEYPOINT: Normal results: Estrogen levels vary in women, ranging from 24-149 picograms per ml of blood. In men, the normal range is between 12-34 picograms per ml of blood.

Progesterone levels vary from less than 150 nanograms per deciliter (ng/dL) of blood to 2,000 nanograms in menstruating women. During pregnancy, progesterone levels range from 1,500-20,000 ng/dL of blood.

Testosterone values vary from laboratory to laboratory, but can generally be found within the following levels:
- Women. 30-95 ng/dL
- Prepubertal children. Less than 100 ng/dL (boys), less than 40 ng/dL (girls)

> **KEYPOINT: Estrogens that a woman normally produces during her reproductive years stimulate a blood protein called sex hormone-binding globulin (SHBG). This protein absorbs and holds any male hormones such as testosterone or DHEA, which circulate in small amounts in all women. These male hormones called androgens will stimulate hair to grow in a male pattern—with beard, mustache and abdominal hair growing up from the pubic area toward the navel (called the Mena or Happy Trail on women)—and stimulate the growth of acne in the skin. When sex hormone-binding globulin is high, it deactivates the androgens so that women do not have these male hair problems or acne. In fact, the birth control pills that decrease acne do so because the estrogen in the pills increases SHBG.**

Also, just before menopause, when the ovaries do not ovulate regularly, estrogen levels drop and androgen levels are freer to stimulate hair growth and acne. That is why most menopausal and some perimenopausal women will notice increased facial hair growth as well.
- **Obesity**—An increase in body weight beyond the limitations of skeletal and physical requirements, as the result of an excessive accumulation of fat in the body.
- **Ovarian/Adrenal Tumors**—Produce androgens and can cause hirsutism. May also be associated with male pattern balding, deepening of the voice, and enlargement of the clitoris.
- **Polycystic Ovarian Syndrome (PCOS)**—An

endocrine disorder, primarily in younger women. The ovaries develop cysts and fail to release eggs. PCOS is a medical condition that is also known as Polycystic Ovaries, Sclerocystic Ovarian Disease, Stein-Leventhal Syndrome, Chronic Anovulatory Syndrome, Polycystic Ovarian Syndrome, and Polycystic Ovarian Disease (PCOD). It is the most common female endocrine (hormonal) disorder and is characterized by multiple abnormal ovarian cysts. Symptoms of PCOS can include excessive weight gain and obesity; irregular, heavy or completely absent periods; ovarian cysts; excessive facial or body hair; alopecia (male pattern hair loss); acne; skin tags (growths from the skin); Acanthosis Nigricans (brown skin patches); high cholesterol levels; exhaustion or lack of energy.

> **KEYPOINT: Two of the most common causes of hirsutism are polycystic ovarian syndrome (PCOS) and idiopathic hirsutism (PCOS is the most common hormonal disorder among women of reproductive age in the U.S). Approximately 70 percent of women with a history of PCOS develop UFH during their teens or early 20s.**

Elevated levels of male hormones may occur with PCOS, causing terminal hair growth on the face, chest, lower abdomen, back, arms and legs. Medications commonly used to counter the UFH caused by excess androgen are spironolactone (Aldactone), finasteride (Propecia, Proscar) and flutamide (Eulexin). Vaniqa® is also commonly recommended.

- **Post Menopause**—An estimated 70 percent of postmenopausal woman who are not taking hormone replacement therapy will develop UFH, with changes in the androgen-to-estrogen ratio.
- **Pre/Post Pregnancy** brings on a wide variety of skin

conditions which require some assistance. Acne can surge, melasma (pregnancy-induced hyper-pigmentation) begins, various pruritic (itchy) skin rashes occur, and a host of other skin-related problems materialize, as well as UFH and UBH.

- **Pregnancy**—Pregnancy and childbirth can initiate hormone changes, giving rise to UFH.
- **Puberty**—For some young women, development of terminal hair at puberty (such as those of the eyebrows, scalp and pubic area) appears on the face.
- **Stimulation**—In many cases, when we are young girls and we notice hair growth, we immediately start to pluck, wax, shave or do anything else we can think of! Contrary to popular belief, shaving does not literally cause "more" hair growth. On the other hand, plucking does agitate the base of the hair follicle and can actually stimulate hair regrowth. Other forms of professional hair removal, if done *incorrectly*, can also stimulate regrowth. So remember, before you start to remove hair, educate yourself on the possible repercussions. This is also important to teach to young girls as well. *See Chapter 7 for details on all forms of hair removal.*

**KEYPOINT: It is difficult to determine for sure which method of hair removal will agitate or stimulate your hair follicles (on a individual level). If you notice UFH or UBH, consult a physician or hair-removal professional to discuss your options for PERMANENT HAIR REDUCTION to avoid creating a really "hairy" problem. This is especially important for very young girls.
(See Chapter 11 for more details on preteens and teens.)**

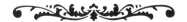

CHAPTER 7

TREATMENT OPTIONS

"The journey of a thousand miles begins with one step."
—Lao-Tse

The treatment of hirsutism will depend upon the underlying cause. If there is truly a "disorder," a patient will require a form of Systemic (Medicinal or Hormone) Therapy to treat the disorder. Natural Hormone Therapy may also be an option in some cases. Medical therapy is successful in preventing new hair growth, but does not affect existing hair. Due to this fact, in most cases patients will also require a form of Cosmetic Therapy to reduce and/or remove the existing hair.

In order to prevent further growth AND remove existing hair, the best treatment option is a combination of systemic and cosmetic treatment plans (see *Combination Therapy* in Chapter 19 for details).

The goals of treatment, in general, are to:

- Address any serious underlying medical conditions.
- Slow down or stop new hair growth.
- Remove, reduce or camouflage the existing hair.
- Address any related health problems, such as menstrual irregularities.
- Anticipate any associated long-term health conditions, such as cardiovascular disease.

> **KEYPOINT: Before prescribing any treatment, your doctor will carefully assess your degree of hirsutism so that the effectiveness of treatment can be gauged over time.**

A) Systemic and Medicinal Therapy

Systemic Therapy (or hormone therapy) always requires a year or more of treatment for maximal benefit. Long-term treatment is frequently required as the problem tends to recur when treatment is stopped. The patient must therefore be an active participant in the decision to use systemic therapy and must understand the rare risks as well as benefits.

Once you are properly diagnosed, the physician will prescribe a treatment plan. Once the treatment has proven to be effective, it is continued indefinitely.

> **KEYPOINT: Because it is usually not possible to cure the hormonal problem causing the excess hair growth, hirsutism will return if medical treatment is stopped.**

The hirsutism of PCOS and idiopathic hirsutism are treated in similar ways. The treatment of PCOS may further involve treatment of infertility, diabetes and risk factors for cardiovascular disease. Several methods of hair removal, reduction or lightening can be used in conjunction with medication to offer better results (this is combination therapy—see Chapter 19). Women with hirsutism who are trying to conceive or are already pregnant cannot take medications used to treat hirsutism, and should ask their doctors about the safety of the various mechanical and chemical treatment methods during pregnancy.

Several medications are available for the treatment of hirsutism. These medications can decrease the distribution of body hair, halt the growth of new hair, and decrease the growth rate and coarseness of existing hair. Most of these medications must be taken for at least six months before improvement is detectable, and not all medications are equally effective in all women.

> **KEYPOINT: The medicinal treatment options mentioned below are strictly for reference only. Please consult your physician in order to be properly diagnosed and treated.**

Several medicines can alter the impact of androgen hormones on the body and skin. Here are some of the more common prescribed medicines used to treat hirsutism:

1) Anti-Androgen Medicines: Directly decrease androgen production or block the action of androgens on the hair follicle. Because these medications may cause birth defects, doctors usually also prescribe oral contraceptives for sexually active women. There are many anti-androgen medicines available; consult with your physician about all options, risks and side effects. It is unsafe to take anti-androgen medicines during pregnancy. A few of the more common anti-androgen medicines are:

- **Spironolactone** (Aldactone)—This is the most commonly used medicine to treat hirsutism. It blocks the effect of androgens on the hair follicle. It is often used together with birth control pills. Spironolactone is usually prescribed if a six-month trial of oral contraceptives does not reduce hirsutism. Between 60 and 70 percent of women with hirsutism will notice improvement when taking spironolactone. If the initial dose is not effective after several months of treatment, your doctor may recommend a higher dose.

- **Cyproterone Acetate** is an anti-androgen but is also a teratogenic and a weak glucocorticoid and progestogen. Given continuously it produces amenhorrhea (absense of menstruation), and so is normally given for days 1 to 14 of each cycle. In women of childbearing age, contraception is essential.

- **Finasteride** may be as effective as spironolactone in some women with hirsutism. It is not approved for use in women in the United States, but is available as a medication for male pattern balding (Propecia) or prostate cancer (Proscar) in men. However, many insurers will not cover the costs of finasteride for cosmetic reasons in either women or men.

- **Cyproterone Acetate** reduces hirsutism in about 70 percent of women, but is currently unavailable in the United States. It is used commonly in Europe and Canada, where it is a component of a type of birth control pill.

- **Metformin**—A medication that is commonly used for the treatment of type 2 diabetes (adult-onset). However, it is also sometimes used for women with polycystic ovarian syndrome (irregular periods and hirsutism or acne) to help make periods more regular and possibly improve fertility. Some women also note some improvement in their hirsutism with metformin, but it does not appear to be as effective as the other medications mentioned above.

2) Corticosteroids (Steroids): Used to treat a rare chronic condition called Congenital Adrenal Hyperplasia.

3) Oestrogens (e.g. **Oral Contraceptives/Birth Control Pills**): Oral contraceptives alter levels of several hormones, including androgens. Oral contraceptives alter levels of several hormones, including androgens. They are usually the first choice and the most commonly used medication to treat hirsutism. Between 60 and 100 percent of women with hirsutism will notice improvement when taking these medications. Oral contraceptives can also help establish regular menstrual cycles in women with hirsutism who have irregular cycles or who do not menstruate at all. One new pill, *Yasmin,* has become popular with many women for the treatment of hirsutism. However, it has not been shown that Yasmin is any more effective than other birth control pills. Oral contraceptives can cause side effects such as high blood pressure and high cholesterol levels. Therefore, your doctor may order tests before prescribing them. Combined pills, which contain a non-androgenic progestogen (e.g. *Dianette* or *Marvelon*) have a theoretical advantage over older combined pills, and will result in a slow improvement in hirsutism in a majority of cases. They should normally be used first, unless there is a contraindication. Other combination birth control pills (containing both estrogen and progesterone) can counterbalance the masculine effects of androgen hormones and decrease the production of testosterone by the ovaries. Hirsutism may improve after 6 to 12 months of consistent use of birth control pills.

4) Other: There are other agents of doubtful efficacy, including bromocriptine and cimetidine. Also, Flutamide is a new agent which remains to be fully evaluated.

> **KEYPOINT: For continued updates on therapies you can frequently check the following Web site: www.uptodate.com**

****

B) Natural Hormone Therapy (Bio-Identical Hormone Replacement Therapy): See Chapter 8

****

C) Cosmetic and "At Home" Hair Removal

This book is a tool to help you understand hair growth better so you can learn what the best *plan of action* is for your particular situation. Every person is unique; therefore, your treatment plan should be tailored to fit your specific needs.

In my practice (Divine Laser Hair Removal., Inc.), I chose to work with IPL (Intense Pulsed Light), and I am very happy with the short- and long-term results. Since I am experienced with IPL, I tend to be partial to Intense Pulsed Light (IPL) and combination therapy treatments, which you will learn more about in the following chapters.

I know this is repetitive, but you must treat the disorder

first (if applicable) with systemic/medicinal therapy and then treat the actual "hairiness" from a cosmetic standpoint. If you do not complete a thorough treatment plan, you will wind up just camouflaging and compounding the problem. I have seen it happen too many times. Women just surrender to being "hairy" and suffer medical consequences down the road. This book was written to help women understand that there may truly be a medical reason to their hairiness that can be detrimental to their health.

On the flip side, your hairiness may not be a medical condition from a disorder. All you may need is cosmetic therapy but not all patients are candidates for IPL or laser treatments. Therefore, I wanted to include a list of alternate hair removal/reduction options (other than my first choice of IPL) in order to offer something for everyone and cover all bases and options for _ALL_ people.

> **KEYPOINT: Be aware that to some degree, hair follicles can be easily stimulated as well. It is important to understand that in the process of trying to permanently reduce hair, the opposite can occur, especially if treatments are performed in a poor manner or if settings used in certain treatments (like electrolysis or laser and IPL) are too low. Certain forms of temporary removal can actually stimulate growth. The bottom line: BE CAREFUL when choosing a method of hair removal.**

Only a mere eight percent of women rely strictly on the superior technology and expertise of licensed professionals to perform hair removal procedures. Spas, salons and specialty clinics offer waxing/sugaring, electrolysis, IPL and laser hair-removal techniques. Waxing and sugaring techniques are fairly simple. Typical costs for professional waxing run from $10 to $75. Electrolytic and laser techniques permanently remove hair from *effectively treated follicles and are more costly.* These highly sophisticated technologies are widely used in the industry, and their effectiveness is rapidly evolving.

KEYPOINT: IPL/laser treatment is my first choice when it comes to cosmetic options. The options mentioned below are just for reference and include treatments OTHER than laser or IPL. Check with your physician to make sure you are a candidate for some of the more professional options.

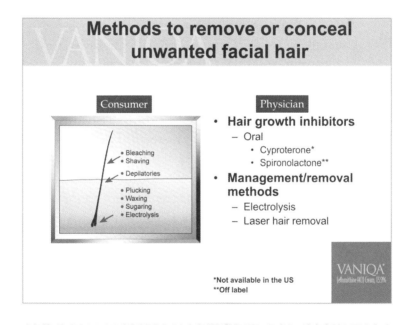

KEYPOINT: 43 percent of women are not satisfied with their current removal method mainly due to: INCONVENIENCE, BOTHER, TIME SPENT REMOVING, TREATING AND CONCEALING, PAIN, IRRITATION.

Here is a breakdown of cosmetic methods:

- **Bleaching**: A cream that is applied to the hair to turn hair a pale, skin-matched shade. Women have used bleach to lighten fuzzy upper lips for years. You should always test a bit of commercial hair bleach on a small area of your arm before using it on your upper lip hair, just to make sure it won't irritate your skin.

  Pros: It is quick, easy, inexpensive and painless, and kits are readily available at drugstores and grocery stores.

  Cons: Applying bleaching creams can be messy, and many people dislike the odor. If you have sensitive skin, you might have an allergic reaction to the chemicals which may cause a rash or inflammation, and the results are very temporary. Bleaching creams may not be as effective on people with coarse hair and can sometimes actually ENHANCE the appearance of thicker hairs (especially in the sunlight).

- **Burn It Off**: This is not a common form of removal, but essentially you take a lighter and quickly pass it over the area that you wish to remove the hair. The hair is singed and you just wipe it away.

  Pros: Inexpensive, leaves skin soft (although temporarily) and works very quickly.

  Cons: Results are temporary, and the process can be very dangerous for obvious reasons. Many people dislike the harsh odor of burning hair.

- **Depilatories**: A depilatory is a cream or liquid that removes hair from the skin's surface. Depilatories work by reacting with the protein structure of the hair, so the hair dissolves and can be washed or wiped away. You can use a chemical depilatory cream to remove hair anywhere on the body, except around nipples or eyes.

Pros: It is quick, easy, inexpensive and painless, and kits are readily available at drugstores and grocery stores. They're best on the leg, underarm, and bikini areas; special formulations may be used on the face and chin.

Cons: Applying depilatories can be messy, and many people dislike the odor. If you have sensitive skin, you might have an allergic reaction to the chemicals in the depilatory, which may cause a rash, burning sensation or inflammation. Depilatories may not be as effective on people with coarse hair. The results are very temporary.

- **Electrolysis**: This is truly the one true form of "permanent hair removal" (if it is performed perfectly, which is extremely difficult to accomplish). Electrolysis destroys the ability of the follicles to grow hair by using electricity to generate heat within the hair follicles. Electrolysis has become less popular than laser treatment because it is more likely to leave small areas of scarring and is tedious to perform. Electrolysis can destroy all hair colors and is successful on most skin types. However (yes, there is a big however), it is a very difficult procedure to master. I consider it an art form; it takes a true "artist" to achieve results. A fine needle is inserted into every follicle, one by one. I am a certified electrologist and I practiced for over three years. I can speak firsthand about the difficulty level. The needle must be inserted at a perfect angle and at the exact depth in order to emit the electrical pulse and destroy your target. If you hit or poke through the walls of the follicle or bypass the root, it is quite painful and can cause bleeding and scarring, as well as possibly stimulate hair growth instead of destroying the follicle. Each hair must also be in an "anagen phase" (growth phase) in order to destroy it, so many treatments are required to achieve this. A small area such as the upper lip may take a total of 4 to 10 hours, and a larger area such as the bikini line may take 8 to 16 hours.

There are three modalities of electrolysis. They all are similar in the fact that a sterile metal needle is slid into the hair follicle. The difference in modalities is the type of electrical current used.

Thermolysis is what most people think of when they think of electrolysis. A small alternating current is applied. This cauterizes the follicle. This current only goes to the target, the base of the follicle.

Galvanic is when direct current is applied. Your body will use its own salts and fluids to make galvanic lye within the follicle, destroying it chemically. Direct current flows throughout your body and out into a ground that you hold. You do not feel it flow through, but because it does, there are certain contraindications such as pregnancy, pacemaker, implanted electrodes, epilepsy, metal pins or rods in the body.

The Blend—The third modality is actually a combination of the other two and is called The Blend. They compliment each other; if there is heat, fewer chemicals are needed, and if there are chemicals, less heat is needed. Your electrologist will determine which modality to use.

I believe there is still a "niche" for electrolysis. I personally recommend electrolysis only for the following reasons:

• Small areas or areas with a minimal amount of hairs.

- Areas that laser/IPL cannot treat (like eyebrows).
- For blond, true red, gray or white hairs.
- As a "grand finale" to (or in conjunction with) laser or IPL treatments. *You may be left with a few random hairs spread over large areas like legs or arms after a group of laser or IPL treatments. It can be easier to use electrolysis in order to target and treat these specific hairs to achieve an overwhelmingly smooth ending!

Contraindications for Electrolysis

- Collagen injections in area to be treated.
- Tendency to develop keloid scars.

> **Pros:** Electrolysis is the only type of hair removal that can claim permanent hair "removal" (as opposed to permanent hair reduction from laser and IPL treatments). Works on all hair colors and skin types.

> **Cons:** Electrolysis takes big bucks and lots of time, so it's usually only used on smaller areas such as the upper lip, eyebrows and underarms. Many people describe the process as painful, and dry skin, scabs, scarring and inflammation may result after treatment. Infection may be a risk if the needles and other instruments aren't properly sterilized. It is a very difficult procedure to perform, and if done incorrectly, treatments can be completely ineffective.

- **Shaving**—Using a razor, a person removes the tip of the hair shaft that has grown out through the skin. Some razors are completely disposable, some have a disposable blade, and some are electric. Guys often shave their faces, and women often shave their underarms, legs and bikini areas. Shaving is a safe and effective method for hair removal, but may require daily sessions. Believe it or not, shaving does not make the hair grow back quicker or coarser. If shaving somehow did increase hair growth, you can be sure that we'd know about it, because it would essentially be a cure for male pattern baldness. Billions of dollars are spent every year by men trying to regrow their hair. If all they had to do was shave it for a while, you'd be seeing a lot more shiny domes in the short term.

KEYPOINT: All hair growth takes place in the hair follicle, which is below the skin. When we cut or shave our hair, we're cutting the dead part of it that has grown out past the surface of the skin. This doesn't affect hair growth in any way, neither positively nor negatively.

Pros: All you need is some warm water, a razor, and if you choose, shaving gel or cream. You don't need an appointment, shaving is a do-it-yourself endeavor, resulting in smooth, hairless skin.

Cons: Can cause pseudofolliculitis (razor burn), bumps, nicks, cuts and ingrown hairs. Ingrown hairs occur when hairs are cut below the level of the skin. When the hair begins to grow, it grows within the surrounding tissue rather than growing out of the follicle. The hair curls around and starts growing into the skin, and irritation, redness and swelling can occur at the hair follicle. The result is *very* temporary, and shaving large areas (like full legs) can be extremely time-consuming.

- **Sugaring**: This hair removal method relies on a sugar compound which can be purchased at most drugstores. Sugaring is very similar to waxing and produces the same results, but does not require as much heating.

- **Threading**: This is an ancient technique popular in countries such as Iran or Egypt. The procedure utilizes a piece of cotton thread which is twisted and pulled along the area of unwanted hair, lifting hair directly from the follicle. The pain is similar to tweezing and waxing. Commonly used for eyebrow shaping.

  Pros: Completely removes hair with less irritation than waxing because the thread pulls only at the hair and saves the skin. It is also a fairly quick and clean procedure (unlike waxing, which can be quite messy). The process is very precise and offers very nice, neat results when sculpting eyebrows.

  Cons: Not easily available because it is not a common practice. It can also be more expensive than waxing. You cannot do this yourself, so you must find a professional to do it. Like plucking, it can stimulate hair growth, and hair can return coarser and darker.

- **Tweezing/Plucking**: Using tweezers, a person stretches the skin tightly, grips the hair close to the root, and pulls it out. This method may backfire, however. Plucking can irritate the base of the hair follicle and may stimulate hair regrowth.

  Pros: It is inexpensive because all you need are tweezers, and since you pull the hair form the root, it can take a while to regrow.

  Cons: Plucking is time-consuming because you can only remove one hair at a time. It can be painful, so it's best to do it only on small areas, such as the eyebrows, upper lip and chin. If the hair breaks off below the skin, a person may get an ingrown hair. After plucking, you may notice temporary red bumps (follicular edema) because the hair follicle is swollen and irritated. *Plucking can stimulate hair growth and hair can return coarser and darker and also cause scarring and skin discoloration.

KEYPOINT: I do not recommend this form of hair removal at all. It is negative on so many levels. Also, plucking will interfere with permanent results if you are getting laser, IPL or electrolysis treatments.

- **Waxing**: A sticky wax is spread on the area of skin where the unwanted hair is growing. A cloth strip is then applied over the wax and quickly pulled off, taking the hair root and dead skin cells with it. The wax can be warmed or may be applied cold. Waxing can be done at a salon or at home. It removes hair for a period of time ranging from one to three weeks without producing stubble. With the exception of hair that has been hormonally stimulated, hair that is waxed may grow back fine or sometimes finer.

  Pros: Waxing leaves the area smooth and is long-lasting. Waxing kits are readily available in drug-stores and grocery stores. Hair regrowth looks lighter and less noticeable than it is after other methods of hair removal, such as shaving.

  Cons: Many people mention that the biggest drawback to waxing is the pain when the hair is ripped out by the root. A person may notice tem-porary redness, inflammation and bumps after waxing, and it is tough on the skin in general. Professional waxing is also expensive compared to other hair removal methods. It can also be messy (especially if you try it at home).

> **KEYPOINT:** People with diabetes should avoid waxing because they are more susceptible to infection. Also, teens who use acne medications such as tretinoin and isotretinoin may want to skip the wax because those medicines make the skin more sensitive. Patients with moles or skin irritation from sunburn should also avoid waxing. Waxing will interfere with permanent results if you are getting laser, IPL or electrolysis treatments and should be avoided.

D) Other

- **Vaniqa®** (See Chapter 17)

- **Weight Loss**: In overweight women, losing weight can decrease levels of androgens and lessen hirsutism. Women with menstrual irregularities may also notice that their cycles become more regular after they lose weight.

E) Treatment of the Rare Causes of Hirsutism

The treatment of most of the rare causes of hirsutism is targeted at the underlying condition; hirsutism may lessen or resolve with effective treatment. Hormone-secreting tumors can be surgically removed and may require additional chemotherapy or other medications.

F) Ultimate Treatment Option: Combination Therapy—Healing You From the Inside Out. (See Chapter 19.)

CHAPTER 8

NATURAL HORMONE THERAPY:
Bio-identical Replacement Therapy
for Men and Women

(Check www.sottopelletherapy.com for more information about
Dr. Tutera and this remarkable therapy)

**"Doubt is a thief that often makes us fear to
tread where we might have won."**

—William Shakespeare

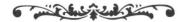

This treatment option deserved its own chapter! I know because I am a happy patient! Bio-identical hormones are completely natural and are slipped painlessly under the skin in your hip. *Although this option was a good choice for me, it may not be right for everyone. Do your research first!*

The information below is from the SottoPelle® Center for Hormonal Balance and Well Being: Dr.Gino Tutera, M.D., F.A.C.O.G., Medical Director in Scottsdale, Arizona (and is also the medical director for my medical spa Divine Laser Hair Removal, Inc.). This type of therapy has been my choice for help from PMS and Menopausal symptoms. I am personally going through menopause and I did a lot of research and found this therapy to be my best option. I believe it is nothing short of a miracle and I am so thankful I found this method. *Please research similar methods in your area as the information may vary.*

Natural, Hassle-free Hormone Therapy

Are you tired of being tired? Cranky about everything and nothing? Can't think straight; can't remember; can't even get a good night's sleep? If it isn't the hot flashes, then it's the night sweats. And don't even go to the sex drive place! What's that?

If this describes your midlife days and nights, you are probably going through menopause, or andropause (male menopause). This means the production of hormones-the ones that used to keep you so perfectly in balance-has slowed to a trickle. Your body is aging.

The good news? You can still do something about it. You just need to replace what's missing.

SottoPelle® was designed to do just that—to replace the estrogen and testosterone that are so key to your well-being. We're not talking *synthetic pharmaceuticals.* SottoPelle® pellets are manufactured from the highest quality botanical ingredients available and specifically formulated to identically match what your body once produced. No horse urine. No fillers. Just pure, natural, biologically identical hormones-plain and simple.

Easy ? Safe ? Effective

Forget the pills, the patches, the injections and all the rest. SottoPelle® uses the most convenient and effective delivery method available: subcutaneous hormone pellets which are implanted beneath the skin in less than a minute, painlessly. Haven't heard about pellets? It may surprise you to know that bio-identical pellets have been used successfully by patients throughout Europe and the United States since the 1930s. And study after study has proven them to be not only safe, but beneficial to the health of those using this method of hormone replacement. IF it seems too good to be true, see for yourself. Order a copy of *You Don't Have to Life with It; Uncovering nature's power with SottoPelle® bio-identical hormones,* by Gino Tutera, M.D., F.A.C.O.G., founder of SottoPelle®. You'll wonder why you haven't heard about SottoPelle® sooner.

Naturally, Every*body* Prefers SottoPelle®

It's amazing what something this simple can do. The pellets deliver a steady, low dose of natural estrogen and testosterone that flows directly into your blood steam whenever your body needs it. After your first treatment, you'll be astonished as a *new you* begins to emerge. And another thing-there is few if any, side effects other than health benefits. Research on depression, weight gain, osteoporosis, prostate cancer and breast cancers shows that bio-identical pellet therapy demon-strates positive impacts in all of these areas.

The best news of all: SottoPelle® pellets last 4 to 6 months, making this therapy so hassle-free, you'll forget you're even on any type of hormone replacement.

> **KEYPOINT: You can purchase a book by Gino Tutera, M.D., F.A.C.O.G. called You Don't Have To Live with It, Uncovering nature's power with SottoPelle bio-identical hormones on his websitewww.sottopelletherapy.com.**

The following is reprinted with the express permission of SottoPelle®. This information is relevant because in many cases, hormonal disturbances can cause abnormal hair growth.

A) YOU MAY HAVE A HORMONE PROBLEM IF:

- Your husband happens to look at you the wrong way, and you end up in tears
- During dinner someone asks you to please pass the salt, and you start sobbing uncontrollably
- Your bathroom scale tells you, you've gained a pound since yesterday and you kick your cat down the stairs
- You live in a nice house with a great family amidst financial security and you feel your life is going to hell in a hand basket
- You always thought, "life begins at 40", and when you get there you see nothing but dead end signs
- Your boss tells you shortly after lunch that you should probably take the day off and go home and soak in a hot bath….and the office applauds
- You have lost your "life" as you once lived it.
- You have lost your ability to enjoy life!
- The thought of driving your car a few blocks makes

you nervous and break out in a cold sweat while having a hot flash
- Your friend says you may have a hormone problem, and you take her off your Christmas card list
- Your over 50, and you think you don't have a hormone problem- you may have a hormone problem

B) *What does Bio-identical mean?*

Bio-identical means that the structures of the hormones are exactly the same as the ones produced by the human body. Bio-identical hormones are not synthetic simulations or replicas. They are made from soy and natural plant-based ingredients and possess the exact hormonal structure of human hormones.

C) *What is Bio Identical SottoPelle® Hormone Therapy used for and how does it work?*

For women, traditional hormone replacement therapies default "to a trials and error" method of trying to find the right combination of estrogen and testosterone dosages that will bring you back to something resembling normality.

SottoPelle® hormone pellet therapy works in unison with your body. It is the only form of hormone delivery that allows the body to take and receive estrogen and testosterone directly into the blood stream, as well as, control the release of these hormones according to the body's needs. As an example when you need more as in exercise and less when you need less as in when you are sleeping.

However, most of the time, it seems that you are supposed to settle for and adjust to a new set of realities….ones for which you never bargained. These may include:

- A roller coaster effect of up and down emotions and mood swings
- Depression
- A diminished (or even nonexistent) sex drive
- Night sweats and hot flashes
- Headaches
- Lack of motivation to do things you enjoyed
- A lack of energy
- Chronic fatigue
- Anxiety
- Irritability & anger
- Mental "fuzziness"
- Inability to focus or concentrate
- A permanent, daily regimen of pills
- Think you have Attention Deficit Disorder
- Coordinating the timing of the pills' peak impact with desired activities.
- Loss of muscle mass; lack of physical endurance
- Osteopenia or osteoporosis

But it doesn't have to be that way!

After securing a set of blood tests for verifying your current levels of hormones, the pellets are inserted under the skin in the office, a total of 5 minutes, and your new life begins. After taking so many pills for so long, it may seem almost impossible that just a few rice sized pellets can actually provide all that your body needs. Because the pellets are not in ingested into your stomach, then processed by your liver, many of the flavorings, buffers, and "excess medicine" are not required. When your body is low on either estrogen or testosterone, it seeks a source for those, finds what it needs from the pellets and processes and applies it immediately. Women using pellets are:

- *Feeling much more in control of their bodies and their lives*
- *Sleeping more consistently and soundly*
- *More interested in sex*
- *Enjoying renewed vitality and zest*
- *Realizing greater mental clarity*
- *More enthusiastic*
- *Calm, relaxed and stable*
- *They are in complete control of the release of their hormones, unlike pills, creams, suppositories, and injections which control you.*

BIO-IDENTICAL HORMONES in SottoPelle® Pellets CAN ALSO:

- Can decrease Body fat
- Can give you relief from depression and anxiety
- Can increase energy, mental focus and sexual drive
- Work in partnership with your body 24/7
- Have few if any side effects and are hassle-free
- Last up to 6 months

KEYPOINT: This therapy is also recommended for men.
Why SottoPelle® Therapy for Men?

Hormonal needs for men have received national attention, but with marginal treatment options available. Hormonal treatments for men can be expensive, require daily consumption, and in many cases, need to be carefully timed with their partner's needs for normal sexual activities and pleasure.

SottoPelle® Therapy as administered by Dr. Tutera is the *only* method of testosterone therapy that gives sustained and **consistent testosterone levels** throughout the day, for 4 to 6 months, without any "roller coaster" effect. *Other forms of testosterone therapy simply cannot deliver such steady hormone levels.* Dr. Tutera has achieved excellent results treating men with **SottoPelle® therapy**. In fact, there have been **no major side effects** in the entire history of this type of therapy and few if any minor side effects.

Men & Andropause

Current medical research now defines a male equivalent to menopause referred to as *andropause.* Men experience a more gradual decline in hormone levels. They lose approximately one percent of their testosterone and 2.5 percent of their DHEA per year beginning at age 30.

Men find themselves lacking in sexual desire, gaining weight, losing muscle mass and feeling sluggish, depressed and irritable. Yet, they believe they must endure these body and hormonal changes as part of aging.

Testimonials:

"I have been using SottoPelle® therapy since 2000. I have never felt so good- my anxieties have disappeared, I have more energy, my hair and skin are better. I feel happy and calm. Thank goodness for Dr. Gino Tutera."

—Keely Smith, celebrity and singer

"I love the SottoPelle® bio-identical natural hormones! With history of cancer in my family, I feel safer and wouldn't even consider synthetic hormones. My headaches are gone, I don't' have crying spells anymore, my libido has improved, and I am finally losing those extra pounds I put on!"

—Pam Scott

"Thank you for saving my life—my marriage & for giving me back my energy and self worth. You told me you could make me feel 35 again—I feel 500% better and you were wrong about the feeling 35. I feel 25!

Thank you,
Bonnie

"After years of mood swings and tears trying every natural remedy to avoid synthetic hormones…I am truly myself again! I am so glad I found this therapy and Dr. Tutera. I live 3 hours away and the trip here is worth every minute I spend on the road"

"Believe me; I was shocked when my blood test revealed I had zero testosterone. With SottoPelle my energy level is higher than the young people I work with and my memory is sharper. It is rare to find such a compassionate doctor these days. Thank you for the comfort we feel from you and your staff.

"I have been using SottoPelle therapy since 2000. I have never felt so good. My anxieties have disappeared; I have more energy, my hair and skin is better. I feel happy and calm. Thank goodness for Dr. Gino Tutera."

"Although I am only 38 years old, I feel like 20 again. I have so much more energy and am happier. Thank you for changing my life for ever."

"Today I visited the office to get my pellet therapy and once again I am amazed at the changes in my life. When I first came to you in 1994, I was woman ready to do anything to stop the terrible PMS symptoms I was experiencing. I remember being almost in a state of war with attitude. I was very abrupt with you, asking for whatever you could give me to stop the feeling of being a pressure cooker. You gently guided me to the less severe choice of therapy, suggesting I may not be so happy with the heavier pharmaceuticals. You held my health and well being in your hands and I am so thankful today that you cared enough to do so. It has been a few years now that I have been on the pellets, estrogen testosterone and the sub-lingual progesterone. Each time I receive them I am reminded of what life was like before. I was a woman lost to love and not even aware of it. Today, once again the tears were right at the surface, my gratitude with you always. When I think I may have past my whole life in that state, never to know passion, I cannot begin to say enough prayers for you. If this is what gets us to heaven, mine will cover you."

CHAPTER 9

THE INTERNAL WAR: PSYCHOLOGICAL AND EMOTIONAL AFFECTS

"Nobody can make you feel inferior without your consent."
—Eleanor Roosevelt

How Do You See Yourself?

If you ask me right now, at this moment in time, the philosophical question, "How Do You See Yourself?" I would quickly and confidently respond, "I am a strong, powerful, successful woman, mother, wife and businesswoman. I am quite secure and love being the center of attention; I am a go-getter; I enjoy public speaking, modeling and acting; I am slightly anal retentive with a touch of perfectionism, which has allowed me to succeed as well as accept failure; I continue to dream BIG and set goals that I will continue to accomplish; I am sexy, desirable, intelligent and charismatic.

On the flip side, if you asked me the same question 20, 15 or even as recent as 5 years ago, I would have sheepishly answered with simple, negative statements. I would have dreaded having to reflect upon my hideous self. I would have said: introverted, shy, scared of crowds to the point of having panic attacks, paranoid, unsuccessful, socially dysfunctional, jealous, unsure of myself, a failure, a high school dropout, the loser in the family, afraid of being alone, feeling I WAS alone, insecure, a follower, ugly, masculine—and did I mention paranoid?!?!

Big change, right? Huge, actually! I have made a complete 180-degree turn since I started laser and IPL treatments, combined with hormone therapy, to reduce my excessive hair growth. This information is so relevant in order to help others understand the impact that unwanted hair growth has on people's views of themselves. Shortly after I started seeing results from my treatments, a completely new person started to emerge. I so badly want to help other women feel this empowering sensation of FREEDOM! UFH and UBH can cause us to have such a negative self-image, and we are blind to the real cause of our distress. We are too scared to strive for our goals, because if we dared to reach them, how would we explain our facial hair? If we were successful, how could we possibly admit to such a beastly problem? It was easier to just sit back and be less than average so nobody would notice us and we would never have to face our deepest demon—HAIR!

How Do You Define Beauty?

Definition of BEAUTY:

1) The quality that gives pleasure to the mind or senses and is associated with such properties as harmony of form or color, excellence of artistry, truthfulness, and originality.

2) A quality or feature that is most effective, gratifying, or telling: The beauty of the venture is that we stand to lose nothing.

American culture is very clear when it comes to defining "beauty." Facial and body hair on women is considered "ugly" or masculine. Our society is very quick to judge the level of hair that is acceptable on a woman. We have created a very vain and appearance-obsessed culture in which certain depictions of "beauty" are embedded in our brains from a very young age. There has never been any type of positive innuendo about women with facial and/or body hair—at least none that I can think of. I can only recall negative connotations such as "The Bearded Woman" or the girl with the "mustache," or how "disgusting" it was when we caught a glimpse of Julia Roberts' unshaved underarm! (I believe "gross" was also used in one of the tabloids). Gross is what is associated with hair on women—period! How can anyone possibly expect a woman who has some hairs on her chin or upper lip not to feel "gross" or inferior when that is exactly what society teaches us? Beauty and the idea of what "beautiful" is simply excludes a woman with any kind of facial or body hair. Many other countries and cultures are far more forgiving of female body hair and openly accept it as a natural, human and sometimes even a sexy characteristic of a woman. Not in America! *This is the LAND OF THE FREE, HOME OF THE SHAVED!*

My "Hair Goggle" Theory

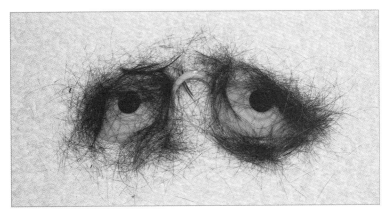

I would like to introduce you to a theory that I have. It is called the "hair goggle" theory. It is similar to the "beer goggle" theory that you may have heard of. It is when the vision of our true self is clouded and distorted because we are subconsciously always looking at ourselves covered in "hair." For instance, you are getting ready for a party. You find the perfect dress, have your hair done, painstakingly apply your makeup, and pamper yourself for days in preparation. Everything should be perfect, but when you take that final look in the mirror, all you can see are those dark hairs on your chin and the red bumps on your neck from tweezing. It completely overshadows the dress and the makeup, and the night is ruined. Of course, in reality, nobody else could even see the hairs on your face because you tweezed and shaved and even bleached them, but you know they are there. You always know, and you can't hide from them. You are constantly wearing "hair goggles."

This distorted vision can even hold us back from pursuing our dreams; reaching our goals; and feeling accomplished and completely successful. I want women around the world to know that they can shed their "hair goggles," put on a pair of Gucci shades and strut their stuff, because we really do have valid, permanent and life-altering options!

Statistics (*Courtesy of SkinMedica, Inc.*)

Only 10 percent of the 22 million women (1 out of every 5 women in the U.S.) who remove UFH weekly or daily consult a doctor about their UFH, and only 4 percent of the same population of women discuss their condition with friends or family members. UFH and UBH are sensitive issues which negatively impact self-esteem. UFH often causes women to feel self-conscious about their appearance, which has lasting effects on their self-image. Women may feel isolated and even guilty about their need to "hide" this "secret." Relationships with friends, coworkers, and family may suffer as a result of the woman's negatively biased self-image. This is why it is so important to offer women with UFH/UBH a **reliable**, effective management plan for dealing with UFH/UBH. Women with UFH are highly motivated to explore and adopt effective means of managing UFH, but sometimes they just need a push. Remember, women with UFH know they have a problem—you don't need to point it out to them. However, they are not always aware that they have options to get rid of it. Sometimes the treatment options need to be pointed out and explained to them.

Also, the condition of excessive hair growth may be intensely distressing, causing discomfort in social situations. In one study, women with hirsutism showed a significant increase in quality-of-life scores when they were asked to re-evaluate their quality of life as if they had no excess facial hair (information courtesy of Skin Medica).

Although it is unrealistic to say that excessive facial or body hair stops women from becoming successful, I definitely believe it is a small (but very relevant) factor. I can say this with confidence because of my own experiences.

My List of "Hairy" Words (*Word Association*)

I sorted through my many interviews from years past and pulled out words that women used to describe themselves. It is basically word association, the primary word being "hairy." I hope this can emphasize the very serious nature of being a hairy woman. These words are very powerful and really put "being hairy" into perspective. This list alone can validate the severity and significance of hirsutism. Even I was surprised by the way some women actually felt about themselves (and I thought I heard it all!). I just think it is sad that so many women are walking around, every single day of their lives, feeling so low about themselves when they don't have to. These words can also be used as "prevention" for parents. As you know, as parents we have a responsibility to listen to what our children are saying (or might be TRYING to say). Young girls suffering from excessive hair growth may give out subliminal messages by using specific words or phrases. They may also exhibit behavior that is unusual. By *listening*, and observing your child very carefully, you can catch the "subliminal" signs early and work on getting your child properly diagnosed and treated. Don't let them suffer—you can prevent years of torment. I just want to scream from the rooftops that THERE IS HELP! *(See the below list of words and phrases)*

Afraid of Intimacy
Afraid to Be touched
Alone
Angry
Annoyed
Antisocial
Anxious (in social situations)
Appalling
Apprehensive
Ashamed
Awkward
Beastly
Bothered
Burdened
Cursed
Demoralized
Depressed
Desperate
Disadvantaged
Disgusting
Dreadful
Embarrassed
Frustrated
Furry
Fuzzy
Gross
Grotesque
Gruesome
Handicapped
Hideous
Horrible
Humiliated
Insecure
Insignificant

Left-Out
Lonely
Manly
Masculine
Misfit
Monstrous
Mortified
Not Feminine
Not Normal
Not Pretty
Not Sexy
Not Worthy
Offensive
On Guard
Oppressed
Outcast
Repulsive
Revolting
Sasquatch
Self-Conscious
Self-Loathing
Timid
Tormented
Ugly
Unacceptable
Unattractive
Uncomfortable
Underprivileged
Undesirable
Unhappy
Unpleasant

CHAPTER 10

MEN AND UNWANTED HAIR

"Men are becoming more and more concerned about
their appearances. This day and age has created
a more "Metro-Sexual" Male.
—Unknown

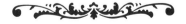

Hirsutism does not only affect the "hairy" person; partners are included in this saga as well. I titled this chapter in dedication to my husband because in my personal story, I was able to pick his brain and get the scoop from a male's perspective. However, I have treated many gay and transgender patients over the years and believe that all partners, male and female alike, suffer consequences as well. Being hairy changes many lives, not just the life of the hirsute person!

It starts out innocent. The partner is completely oblivious and unaware of the condition. As mentioned many times over in this book, we tend to magnify our condition (the "hair goggle" theory). In most cases, the people we initially date do not even notice the hair growth at first. Then, as time passes, our own paranoia can actually force our partners to see the hair. Personally, I started to literally push it into my boyfriends' faces, as if to say, "Here, look at this. Isn't it gross? You can leave me now—go ahead—I am grotesque." Of course, when a relationship actually did fail, I was able to blame it on my hair. I had a legitimate reason for "being dumped" or for why a relationship "just did not work out." Unlike most confused women, I didn't torment myself by sitting around and wondering why he didn't call. I knew immediately: my "hairiness" scared him away!

From another perspective, men can also suffer from excessive and unwanted hair growth (excessive back hair, ear hair, etc.). In turn, they often deal with similar negative issues and affects as well. For instance, how many people point out that guy on the beach with the "hair shirt" and say, "Wow, isn't that sexy?" Not many, I am sure!

Men can also be tormented by the loss of hair on their head and the gain of hair on their ears! I have so many male patients that seek help for the growth of ear hair. It is a very sensitive topic for men. Hair on the ears is difficult to remove both temporarily and permanently due to the contours of the ears. The difficulty is compounded by the color of the hair. Ear hair is often white or gray but laser and IPL cannot kill gray, white or blond hair! In my practice, I came to a stand-still. I couldn't effectively treat the hair on the ears. Luckily, I found Vaniqa®. I now strictly recommend Vaniqa® for ear (and even nose) hair. See Chapter 17 as I detail how Vaniqa® can greatly help alleviate ear hair.

Here are some quotes from a few male patients, as well as husbands, friends and boyfriends of some of my female patients.

❖ Anonymous, Age 39

"My wife is beautiful—absolutely beautiful—but she doesn't see that. She is so paranoid about her face; she does not see anything but the hair. She is so afraid that people will see the stubble or the razor burn, so she cakes on the makeup. I worry about her all the time. I wish she could see what I see."

❖ JJ, Age 27

"My girlfriend recently started laser hair removal treatments, and she is a new person. She suddenly seems so confident, and she is so happy. When I met her, I didn't really care that she was a hairy girl. She has dark hair and light skin so the hairs were pretty noticeable. I never mentioned it to her because I didn't want to embarrass her. One day we were reading the newspaper and there was an ad for a laser clinic in our neighborhood. She asked me if I would go with her on a consultation. I am SO glad she started the conversation because I was able to talk with her about it. She opened up and we talked about it in depth. She told me that she was always afraid to date because if men would see her hair, they would be turned off and break up with her. She was so thankful that I was open-minded about it, and I promised to take her to the consultation and all the treatments and support her completely. She is almost done with the treatments, and she is a different person now."

❖ Anonymous, Age 33

"I always knew my wife had a problem with hair growth, even when I first met her and we were just dating. She was afraid to get intimate in the beginning of the relationship because of it. She had hair on her face, chest, stomach, buttocks and even around her nipples. She was sure I would leave her because of this. She backed away from intimacy for a very long time until I started the dialogue about it. Once she realized that I would listen to her and not get freaked out about it, she was a changed girl. She just needed someone to understand her situation and not judge her. Once she knew that I accepted it, she was a very different person as far as confidence goes, and she became much more open in the bedroom as well. I started doing some research and we finally decided to get laser hair removal. I actually got her a gift certificate for her birthday one year just to get her started. Although I love my wife dearly and always have, the hair did bother me sometimes. Not to the point that I would ever leave her because of it, but I really did not like feeling stubble. It drove me crazy when she would get in bed at night if she didn't shave her legs. It felt like I was sleeping with saguaro cacti. She would shave in the morning and have stubble by the evening, so it was hard to ever get smooth legs. The same was true for the rest of her body. Her face and neck always looked red and irritated from the tweezing, so I helped her find a more permanent solution. She has been done with treatments for a few years now, and I can't explain what an impact it has had on her self-esteem and our relationship. The results are incredible. She doesn't have to shave her legs (or anything else) at all anymore. She has some fine hairs left but they are soft and barely noticeable. We are both thrilled, and there are no more saguaros in the bed!"

❖ Don, Age 30

"My mother has always been very sensitive about her facial hair problem. As kids growing up, my brother and I would catch her shaving her face, and she would cry. I could remember feeling stubble on her face sometimes when she hugged me. When I became an adult, I tried to talk to her about it but she would clam up. One day a girlfriend of mine told me she was going to some place to get laser hair removal treatments. I learned more about it and nonchalantly left a brochure on my mother's countertop when I visited her. She has been going for treatments for months now and she looks awesome! I cannot even believe what this has done for her. She is like a new person. It seems like she laughs more. Maybe it has nothing to do with it, but I really believe it does. She just recently started talking to me about her treatments and how great the results are. I asked her why she didn't get treatments years ago, and she said that she really didn't know much about it and heard that it didn't really work, and she was afraid. I am so glad that I found a facility that cared about her situation and took the time to work with her. I am so happy for her."

❖ Anonymous, Age 22

"I was dating this really nice girl for about two months. One day we were hiking and she was climbing in front of me. I looked up at one point and noticed hair—a lot of hair—on the back of her legs. I couldn't help but cringe. I looked harder and noticed that the hair actually went all the way up her shorts and appeared to cover her buttocks. It freaked me out. I couldn't get past it. Every time I would look at her, I found myself staring and analyzing every part of her. She had hairs on her face and neck and it really turned me off terribly. I really liked her and it upset me to have to break it off with her because she was a great girl. I lied to her and told her that I was getting back with an ex-girlfriend. I still feel bad about it, and this was about two years ago."

❖ Jay, Age 28

"I met a girl in a dance club when I was about 22. We hit it off and danced together and had an awesome time. I kissed her goodnight and held her face in my hands. I felt something weird. I rubbed her face again and realized it was stubble—like real hairy razor stubble. Without realizing it, I blurted out, 'You have something on your face!' She ran off and I never saw her again. Unfortunately, it was just a reaction, but I know now that I hurt that girl so bad. I am married now and love my wife to pieces. She also has some facial hair and body hair. We openly talk about it, and she has been getting laser treatments. I wish I would have had more understanding back then, because ultimately it is no big deal, and apparently a lot of women have it. I am so glad that I didn't judge my wife over this because I would have missed out on the best thing that ever happened to me."

❖ "Smooth-Man," Age 18

"I do not like body hair at all. I shave most of my body; I like to feel smooth and clean. I am finally starting laser hair removal, and after just one treatment, I see good results. Most girls like a smooth chest and stomach. I personally think it looks much better; hair just looks ugly to me. I could never deal with a hairy woman. It is a huge turnoff for me."

❖ Anonymous, Age 46

"I am a hairy dude. Have you seen that movie, *The 40-Year-Old Virgin*? That was me the first time I got waxed. It hurts like hell! I had what they call the 'hair shirt'—my entire front and back was covered in dark, thick hair. You could have combed it. I am so glad my wife started getting laser treatments because she forced me to get a consultation, and I have been hooked ever since. I feel like a new person. I must be 20 pounds lighter since I shed that 'hair shirt.' I love going to the lake now and taking off my shirt without being embarrassed. I swear my wife is more attracted to me, too. She doesn't completely admit it, but she can't keep her hands off me now! It is one of the best things I ever did."

❖ Jim, Age 52

"In my career, I am face-to-face with people on a daily basis, and I like to look well-groomed. My problem is my facial hair, and especially the hair on my ears. I have a very thick beard and I need to shave sometimes twice a day just to look somewhat smooth and presentable. Unfortunately, every single time I shave I get very bad razor burn. I have tried everything. I even went to a dermatologist, and she told me it was called *Pseudofolliculitis Barbae*. She recommended that I try laser hair removal. Some of my hair is gray so I thought I was not a candidate. Luckily, I have a greater percentage of dark hair, so the treatments worked well for me. I still have the white and gray hairs, but the results have been worth their weight in gold. I also became a case study for the clinic and started using Vaniqa® on my ear hair. WOW! I am thrilled! I am so glad that someone took the time to educate me on the process. Otherwise, I would have never tried it and I would still be suffering day after day. Even after the very first treatment, shaving became less of a problem for me. It was like a miracle. I was overwhelmed. I used to get anxiety about shaving, and I would literally dread it. Now, it is such an easy task that I only need to do it two or three times a week (if that). My skin is clearer and people are constantly asking me things like 'Have you lost weight?' or 'What have you done? You look so good.' They can't quite place it, but they can see a difference in my appearance. I also believe it is my new attitude and improved confidence level that people also are responding to. As for my ears, the hair still grows, but it's strange; it hardly comes out. It takes such a long time, I usually forget about it for weeks and then I just shave them and stay pretty smooth for a while. It is so nice not worrying about being close to people! I am one happy camper!"

SEE THE RESULTS FOR YOURSELF:
BEFORE AND AFTER PHOTOS

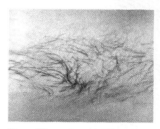

Pre Treatment   Post Treatment

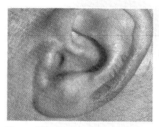
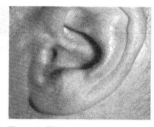

Pre Treatment   Post Treatment

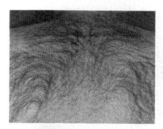
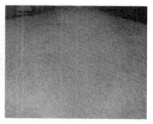

Pre Treatment   Post Treatment

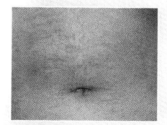
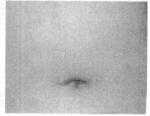

Pre Treatment   Post Treatment

Pictures Courtesy of Palomar Medical Technologies

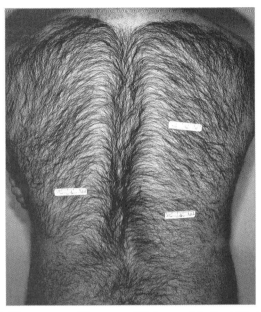

Before IPL Treatments (Coutesy of Palomar Medical Technologies)

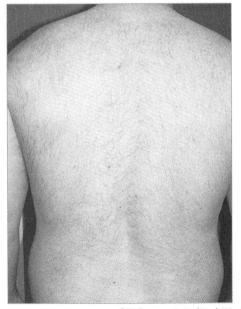

After IPL treatments- courtesy of Palomar Medical Technologies

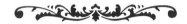

CHAPTER 11

THE PRETEEN AND TEENAGE BATTLE

"The young need guidance and education concerning their bodies; not condemnation, comparisons and criticisms."
—Anonymous

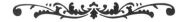

In my search to help other women with this problem I realized that I needed to catch the culprit in the early stages. I wish I had been empowered with knowledge when I was 15 because it would have saved me years of torment. Along my hair-removing journey, I was lucky enough to meet Dr. Tala Dajani, M.D., M.P.H., pediatric endocrinologist and internist at the renowned Phoenix Children's Hospital. I was always searching for a professional in the field that understood my ambitions and shared my passion about this topic. At one point, I almost gave up because most of the doctors I associated with were in the cosmetic industry, and they lacked a deep understanding of the mental toll UFH/UBH takes on people, especially young girls. Most of them were cosmetic surgeons and had little knowledge, and in many cases, little concern about "hair growth." Then I was introduced to Dr Dajani. She was a mirror image of myself, but she had what I didn't—a Ph.D.! We were a perfect fit. I was hands-on, dealing day to day with physically removing the hair with IPL, and Dr. Dajani worked with patients on a clinical level. We would soon come to realize that by combining our experiences and knowledge, we could understand this overwhelmingly significant disorder better than we ever expected to. It was like putting pieces of a puzzle together—finally! Her information and research filled in the blanks for me, and vice versa. It was like we broke a code to a deep, dark secret.

Dr. Dajani refers young female patients to me after careful evaluation and diagnosis. It is important to understand that not all patients (especially very young girls) are candidates for certain types of treatment methods. I also evaluate the clients carefully and recommend a treatment plan. The first step is to make sure the patient is a candidate for permanent hair reduction. There are very specific contraindications (see Chapter 14) that would immediately disqualify a patient. The second step is to evaluate the severity of the problem by getting to know the patient. I never jump into treatments with very young patients. I need to feel confident that they are mature enough to handle the sensation of the treatments as well as the outcome. I am thankful that I have my past experiences to help me gauge these situations. I know how I felt at 16 years old. I remember the trauma and isolation I felt, and I can sympathize with these girls. I also have to build a relationship with the parents because they play an integral part in the success of their child's results. I help educate them on the physical and psychological effects from: (1) dealing with the hair itself, and (2) dealing with the commitment to treatments as well as the pain factor and pre- and post-care requirements. If I feel the effects from the hair growth significantly outweigh the child's (and parents') ability to handle the effects and treatment requirements from the treatments, we are ready to start! Here are some guidelines I use to determine if a young girl is ready for laser/IPL treatments.

> **KEYPOINT: It is important to clearly explain to younger patients (and their parents) that younger patients have a greater amount of dormant follicles. Dormant follicles can (and probably will) produce hair in the future. It is likely that younger patients will need to continue, or at least "maintain," their hair growth with treatments in their future.**

If the answer (for both the child and parent) is yes to the majority of the following questions, I believe the young patient should be capable of handling the treatments. Of course, this is just my own evaluation method that I have created, and it is a general guideline only. All major medical issues have been addressed, and these questions are just to understand the mental and psychological readiness of the patient. I included this chapter because of my experiences as a "hairy" child. I could have saved myself years of anguish if I had received a treatment plan early on. I want this to help parents with young girls suffering from any form of hirsutism to understand that they truly have options and there are professionals that care and can help them as long as they are ready for it. No child should be forced into having treatments; they must WANT to do it for themselves. It is up to the professional offering the treatments to feel comfortable with young girls' decisions. These simple questions have helped me so much in trying to determine what is right for very young patients.

- Is the patient at least 12 years old?
- Did the young patient ASK to get help to get rid of the hair herself?
- Is the young patient distressed about her hairiness?
- Did the parent have to point out the hair growth to the patient or vice versa?
- Does the patient complain about the hair growth?
- Will the parent(s) be able to commit to the treatment plan?
- Will the parents(s) agree to help the patient get to the appointments, help with the pre- and post-care instructions, and support the patient through all stages of the plan for as long as it may take?
- Has the young patient been formally diagnosed with a disorder by a physician? If yes, is she receiving systemic and/or medicinal therapy?
- Does the parent strongly believe the patient is

mature enough to handle the pain and risks involved?

- Is the patient eager and excited to start treatments?
- Did the patient handle the "test spot" treatment adequately from a pain standpoint?

I have treated many young girls over the years and they all are such great role models to me. I adore all of them and greatly admire their courage. One patient in particular has been such a huge inspiration to me. Her name is Andrea and she was 16 when she came to me to get rid of her dark sideburns. I remember how her mom handled the consultation. She was clear in letting me know that Andrea wanted to do something about her sideburns NOT just because a boy broke up with her because of them, but for herself and to make HER more comfortable with her face. The mom was so reassuring and did the best she could to teach Andrea she was a wonderful, bright and beautiful girl with or without the sideburns. It was good to see that Andrea was not broken by having the hair. She was simply ready to get rid of them so other close-minded people would not judge her because of them.

Here are some pictures that Andrea graciously allowed me to use for visual purposes. As you can see in her before picture, her sideburns were quite dark and noticeable. In the "after" picture, there is a great improvement after 3 IPL treatments.

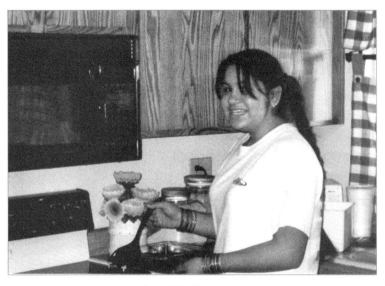

Before IPL Treatments

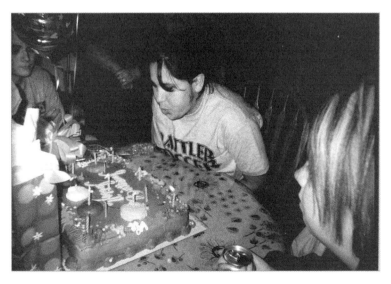

Before IPL Treatments

Laura M. Regan

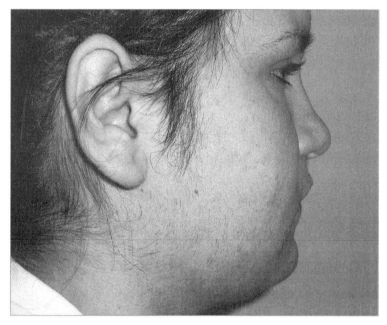

After three (3) IPL treatments

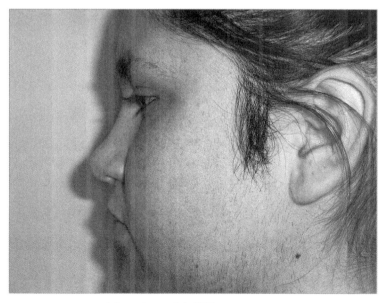

After three (3) IPL treatments

To understand the magnitude of "being young and hairy," from a medical standpoint, I interviewed Dr.Dajani. Here is an excerpt from our discussion:

Why did you become a pediatric endocrinologist?

Dr. Dajani: "I became a physician for two reasons: I was fascinated by the human body and how it worked, and I really enjoy meeting and working with new people. I was trained as a physician at the University of Houston, Texas, medical school. When working with children, teens and young adults, I saw an opportunity to really help shape the health and well-being of a child—the opportunity to start a positive trend that could last a lifetime. While training in internal medicine and pediatrics, I found endocrinology, the study of hormones (chemical messengers in the body), very interesting, and that endocrine problems can be treated with hormone replacement or decreasing excess hormones."

How does "being hairy" emotionally and psychologically affect young girls?

Dr. Dajani: "When girls and young women come to our clinic for evaluation of excess hairiness, they are often quite distraught and limited by the hair. Often, it affects their lives in dramatic ways, limiting them from experiencing and participating in their life's activities fully. At times, these young ladies have developed depression and feelings of worthlessness and helplessness. At times, it is all they think about, and it is hard for them to succeed in school and extracurricular activities. Worst of all, some girls don't experience or enjoy the normal social life of a teenager or young adult and miss out on a very important time in their lives."

What are the most common disorders you diagnose?

Dr. Dajani: "The most common diagnosis is familial or idiopathic hirsutism, meaning that there is no hormone imbalance explaining the excess hair. It is inherited and runs in the family. We also see patients coming in with PCOS."

What do you recommend as far as treatment is concerned?

Dr. Dajani: "Once hair follicles have changed and grow thicker, medical management of hormone imbalances can help prevent new hair follicles from growing, but often don't stop the existing hair. Hair removal and bleaching are modalities to deal with this."

I also interviewed some of my wonderful, lovable young patients that I affectionately call my "hairlings."

❖ Anonymous, Age 16, Facial Hair (lip, cheeks, chin, neck)

"I know other kids stare at me and find me and tease me, especially behind my back. Some days I don't even want to get out of bed or go to school. I stress out about going to parties and stuff like that because if I wax or pluck, I might get bumps and make it worse. It sucks and I hate it. I wish I could get new skin."

❖ T.L., Age 16, Facial Hair

"A boy broke up with me once because he said I had sideburns and he was sick of his friends teasing him about it."

❖ Anonymous, Age 14, Facial Hair and Body Hair

"My mom is always telling me to shave, and I get upset. It seems to bother her more than it bothers me. She even says it in front of my friends and it makes me feel really upset. Now my friends point it out in public and I just want to cry. It's not fair that I have this. My mom has the same thing and she tells me that she went through the same thing when she was a little girl. I just wish there was a cure or something."

❖ Anonymous, Age 15

"I can't dress cool like other girls my age. I am afraid to show my arms, my back and my stomach because of the hair. Every time I bend over, I fear that my shirt will rise up and people will see the hair on my lower back. I am so afraid."

❖ C.K., Age 17

"I just want to be like everyone else. My friends always ask me why I have hair on my face and it hurts my feelings."

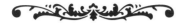

CHAPTER 12

UNWANTED HAIR AND THE TRANSGENDER COMMUNITY

"To be what we are and to become what we are capable
of becoming is the only end of life."
—Robert Louis Stevenson

I have been lucky enough to work with many wonderful people over the years. I have met fascinating people through working in this industry. Many of my patients, colleagues and associates have been true inspirations to me. For the most part, many of these people provided the inspiration for me to write this book. These relationships have taught me a lot, and it was time to share it with everyone. Some of the most inspirational patients have been from the transgender community. I have been privileged to get to know some of these amazing people. I have worked with many patients with *Gender Dysphoria,* including cross-dressers, transgenderists and transsexuals. I have been so touched by their stories. My desire to help them led me to learning more about how to get rid of excessive hair. Although I am neither an expert in this field nor a physician, when it comes to transgender issues, I have educated myself over the years and have a whole new outlook on the community and its struggles. I also accept these people as they are and want to help them. I believe that combination therapy is literally a gift we can give to many of these patients.

I interviewed most of my transgender patients in order to obtain information for this book. I want to share some quotes with you. This can put some things into perspective as far as understanding the significance that hair growth has on their psyche and quality of life.

❖ W.K.S., Age 58

"I am preparing for my surgery, and I have been taking hormones for a long time. Unfortunately, the medications did not get rid of the hair I already had (and I had a very heavy beard). The hair on my face and legs bothers me the most. I feel very alone, and I am afraid of intimacy. I used to get very angry and depressed over this, and I often felt rejected and judged. I have had nine laser treatments and I feel so much better now. The laser treatments made me more confident, and I feel good about myself again. I also use Vaniqa®, and I would highly recommend laser and Vaniqa® treatments to others. I still need a few more treatments, but overall I feel good about laser hair removal and Vaniqa®. I wish I could get it done more often because it helps the overall appearance of my face and neck area, but I have to follow the intervals recommended."

❖ Layla, Age 40, Cross-Dresser

"I am always burdened with facial hair. I have tried everything and nothing has worked. I got severe razor burn, so even when I look my most feminine, it is still very obvious that I am male."

❖ Anonymous, Age 45

"I have been through so much. I was at the end of my rope. I really thought that all my efforts transforming myself were for nothing because of the horrible beard I still have. I had electrolysis for almost two years, but it only seemed to work on certain areas and mostly just thinned it out a little bit. I hated my face. I really did not like looking at it in the mirror sometimes. Now I feel complete. I am on my seventh IPL treatment and I really feel like a new person. I don't hate my face anymore. My skin looks great! I didn't even realize what nice skin I had (even though Laura always points it out). These treatments saved me. I highly recommend it. I also love the Vaniqa® cream. I think that makes my skin look softer, too! The combination of both definitely made the difference. I am almost at the point of not shaving at all, and I finally feel feminine!"

❖ Angelina, Age 29

"I really like the treatments so far. I only had three so far, but I am shaving less and I hardly get razor burn anymore. It is so 'freeing.' I feel like a huge weight has been taken off me. I can't wait for the end result when I have a normal, smooth face."

❖ Anonymous (I used to be Larry), Age 30

"This is all new to me. Not having to shave makes me really feel like a female. I am so happy that I found a place that makes me feel comfortable. Divine Laser has always been very nice and accepting. I felt like Laura really wanted to help me, and she worked extra hard to do it. She used two hand pieces and taught me about combination therapy with Vaniqa®. I am thrilled, to say the least. I wish I had done it years ago!"

❖ D.A., Age 33

"I have been through it all: the hormone therapy and the surgery. I love the outcome, but my true femininity always felt like a step away because of my facial hair. Shaving daily really put a damper on feeling female. As soon as I started my IPL treatments, I knew I made the right decision. I am SO thankful that I found these treatments because I know I would have never felt 100 percent female if I still had a beard. It has taken a lot of treatments, but Laura did explain that it is not an overnight sensation. The key is not giving up. Once I started using the Vaniqa® cream as well as the IPL treatments, the hair just wasn't there anymore. It was like a miracle. It did come back recently, but it is so much thinner and lighter."

****

I believe better results are achieved when patients are understood by their provider. I can relate to many issues that my patients deal with, and the psychological effects must be addressed in order to get results. This is especially true for transgender patients. In many cases, facial and body hair is the final obstacle these patients must hurdle in order to become complete, feminine people. They have often been through so much in their lives, struggling with their identity and fitting into society. Many of my patients have spent so many years evolving into women. They have done everything from surgery to hormone therapy, but are still one small step away from feeling truly feminine. This "small step" is HAIR. They can look feminine and wear the clothes and the makeup, but the stubble on their face reminds them every day that they are not complete (Hair Goggle Theory). Permanent hair reduction is literally life-changing for them. Regular methods of hair removal and reduction are simply not enough to get them the results they need.

KEYPOINT: As a professional, I feel it is my duty to understand all of my patients to the best of my abilities. Learning about gender dysphoria allowed me to treat my patients more effectively.

The excerpts below are from Web sites referred to me by some of my patients. This information is very valuable as it helps laser technicians better understand the magnitude of what these patients are dealing with. As professionals, laser technicians should be as educated as possible about their clientele in order to be able to treat them effectively and fairly.

I found this paragraph from an article written by Douglas K. Ousterhout to be very poignant. It opened my eyes to what these patients go through.

"Feminization of the Transsexual" by Douglas K. Ousterhout, M.D., D.D.S.

"Looking feminine is, of course, extremely important to you. First impressions are often based just upon your face. That which is first seen in an initial contact is frequently what defines you. It establishes not only who you are, but often what sex you are as well. As a transsexual, perhaps nothing is more important to you than appearing sexually the same as you feel emotionally. Facial feminizing surgery can help bring these two together."

Copyright 1994 (1st Revision 1995) Douglas K. Ousterhout, M.D., D.D.S.

http://www.drbecky.com/dko.html

The article speaks about the importance of surgery to complete the transition from male to female. My patients helped me understand that going through the steps to complete surgery and hormonal therapy is such a slow, arduous and often stressful and exhausting process. However, the results can be very positive and lead them in the right direction to truly becoming female. Unfortunately, neither surgery nor hormonal therapy removes or kills the facial and body hair that already exists. My patients are devastated by this because although they worked so hard to become feminine, they are left with the apparent and visible proof that they were born male. I want them to know that there are options for them. They will fight yet another tough battle because it can take many treatments of combination therapy to start to see results. It takes a firm commitment in order for this to work for them. They need to receive treatment from a facility that is familiar with their medical (and emotional) issues.

I also learned about the different types of gender identity issues. This also helped me better understand my patients' specific needs, which ultimately helped us work together to achieve the best possible results.

I found the following information on a website and I am adding it to the book to sum up the information that I feel all professional hair removal facilities should be aware of.

The following information was obtained (verbatim) from a wonderfully informative website—http://www.transgendercare.com

Gender Identity is the last to be identified, and the least understood and researched. Gender identity is one's <u>subjective</u> sense of one's own sex. **Like pain, it is unambiguously felt but is unable to be proven or displayed to others.** One's subjective gender is just as real and tangible as one's physical gender, but unfortunately is not recognized in our culture. When one's **gender identity** does not match one's **physical gender**, the individual is termed Gender Dysphoric. Like minority sexual orientation, gender dysphoria is not pathological, but a natural aberration (departure from the normal), occurring within the population, like blue eyes. As with minority sexual orientation, the percentage of the population having gender dysphoria is in dispute, with estimates ranging between one in 39,000 individuals, and 3 percent of the general population. My experience leads me to feel that the higher figure (3 percent) is closer to the actual prevalence.

Physically male gender-dysphoric individuals have been described, either by themselves or by others, as falling into three distinct groups: **cross-dressers**, **transgenderists** and **transsexuals**.

- **Cross-Dresser**—Those individuals with a desire to wear the clothing of the other sex, but not to change their sex, are termed cross-dressers. Most cross-dressers view themselves as heterosexual men who like to wear women's clothing in private or in public and might even occasionally fantasize about becoming a woman. Once referred to as a transvestite, cross-dresser has become the term of choice.

- **Transgenderist**—Transgenderists are men and women who prefer to steer away from gender role extremes and perfect an androgynous presentation of gender. They incorporate elements of both masculinity and femininity into their appearance. Some persons may see them as male and others may see them as female. They may live part of their life as men and part of their life as women, or they may live entirely in their new gender role, but without plans for genital surgery.

- **Transsexual**—Men and women whose gender identity more closely matches the other physical sex are termed transsexual. These individuals desire to rid themselves of their primary and secondary sexual characteristics and live as members of the other sex. Transsexuals are diagnostically divided into the subcategories of primary or secondary. Primary transsexuals display an unrelenting and high degree of gender dysphoria, usually from an early age (four to six years of age). Secondary transsexuals usually come to a full realization of their condition in their 20s and 30s, but may not act on their feelings until they are much older. Typically, secondary transsexuals first go through phases that would be self-assessed as being a "cross-dresser" or "transgenderist."

While these categories are the generally accepted classifications both within the gender community and among helping professionals, during my work with gender folk I have come to the belief that there is only one cause, one conflict, one condition—but many reactions and adjustments to it. I have gradually come to the conclusion that coming to terms with the conflict between their knowledge of their true gender and their need to be "normal" fosters the same conflict in all gender folk. Because a child's greatest desire is to be normal (like everybody else), the great majority of transgendered individuals create an artificial self which meets this goal. They are often so successful at this that they not only fool everyone else but themselves as well—at least part of the time, in some way.

Once created, physically male gender folk live in their male role—a three-dimensional personality with its own goals, likes and dislikes, values, hobbies, etc. Although indistinguishable from the "real thing," it isn't them. It is an artificial creation for them to be able to *fit in*. This is achieved at the expense of denying—locking away—their natural female selves. (See Brain Gender and Brain Sex.) Their desire to be "normal" has denied them their natural selves. But, as the nagging reality of the deception becomes harder and harder to suppress, they have to express their **true gender** somehow, in some way.

1. **Recognition that one's Brain Gender is different from one's Physical Gender**—This first phase comprises the majority of transgendered persons (75 to 95 percent) and can take the form of seeing one's self as a "woman trapped in a man's body," a need to express one's "feminine side." This stage is mainly concerned with physical/surface changes such as cross-dressing, passing, makeup, wigs, etc. In this first part, many gender folk don't even venture from their own homes in female attire, or they restrict their expression to undergarments (bras, panties) in public. They often have a juvenile (before age 15) and, later, an adult phase. There are often years or decades between the two phases. This level is filled with confusion, conflict, guilt, panic and purging. The so-called "primary transsexual" is an individual who never constructs a male persona and therefore never accepts his male genitals or challenges his female self-map/subjective gender.

2. **Accepting One's True Self**—This stage is much more varied than the first, and has less emotional turmoil. This is the stage where one begins to accept his female self in some way and make lifestyle changes to accommodate this acceptance. One may only accept the need to appear female, still denying his female true self (cross-dresser), or begin to accept his true female self, but concentrating on a superficial physical level of change (transsexual, transgendered).

The self-identified cross-dresser may begin to bring his significant other into his dressing, begin going to cross-dresser meetings and events, or even go out into public. Those individuals more accepting of their true selves will start to look for help in physical transitioning, such as hormones, electrolysis, and surgery, as well as wigs, makeup and clothes.

The major insight lacking at this stage is that they are still under the control of the male persona with all of its unnatural fears, drives, expectations and knowledge. Even their view of their "female selves" is <u>his</u> view, not their freed and autonomous female selves. **They are still trapped in the belief that physical form alone determines gender.**

3. **Becoming One's True Self**—This is the last but unfortunately least experienced part of transitioning. This is the stage when that little girl trapped inside an artificial male persona in order to fit in breaks free, grows up and has her own life—often with markedly different values, temperaments and interests.

It has been my observation that the female self needs little help in growing up and developing if the overpowering weight of the male persona is removed from it. The transgender individual has spent years—decades—developing, reinforcing and living in his male role. Dismantling the male persona takes a great deal of time, effort and outside help. **But an individual's sense of happiness and success is directly parallel with** the degree he has dismantled his male identity, <u>not</u> with his age, physical size, hormones, surgery, etc.

> **KEYPOINT:** According to some of my patients, removing the unwanted facial and body hair is the final step in becoming their true selves. These patients really need to be aware of the great results they can achieve through combination therapy. These patients have come so far and need that final boost of self-esteem that they truly warrant and deserve. In most cases I prefer a combination of hormone therapy, IPL treatments and the daily application of Vaniqa®.

Reasons for Hormone Therapy. Cross-sex hormonal treatments play an important role in the anatomical and psychological gender transition process for properly selected adults with gender identity disorders. These hormones are medically necessary for rehabilitation in the new gender. They improve the quality of life and limit psychiatric co-morbidity which often accompanies lack of treatment. When physicians administer androgens to biological females, and estrogens, progesterone, and/or testosterone-blocking agents to biological males, patients feel and appear more like members of their desired sex.

The Desired Effects of Hormones. Biological males treated with cross-sex hormones can realistically expect treatment to result in: breast growth, some redistribution of body fat to approximate a female body habitus, decreased upper body strength, softening of skin, decrease in body hair, slowing or stopping the loss of scalp hair, decreased fertility and testicular size, and less frequent, less firm erections. Most of these changes are reversible, although breast enlargement will not completely reverse after discontinuation of treatment.

The degree of desired effects actually attained varies from

patient to patient. The maximum physical effects of hormones may not be evident until after two years of continuous treatment. Heredity limits the tissue response to hormones and cannot be overcome by increasing dosage.

Social Side Effects. There are often important social effects from taking hormones, which the patient must consider. These include relationship changes with family members, friends and employers. Hormone use may be an important factor in job discrimination, loss of employment, divorce and marriage decisions, and the restriction or loss of visitation rights for children. The social effects of hormones, however, can be positive as well.

Other Potential Benefits of Hormones. Hormonal treatment, when medically tolerated, should precede any genital surgical interventions. Satisfaction with the hormone's effects consolidates the person's identity as a member of the desired gender and further adds to the conviction to proceed. Dissatisfaction with hormonal effects may signal ambivalence about proceeding to surgical interventions. Hormones alone often generate adequate breast development, precluding the need for augmentation mammaplasty. Some patients who receive hormonal treatment will not desire surgical interventions (information provided by www.symposium.com).

Of course, the hormone therapy is to be administered by their physician and is out of the hands of laser technicians. But this is such a key ingredient for the success of laser and IPL hair reduction. Once the patient has the proper levels of hormones, further hair growth will greatly decrease. This will allow the laser or IPL professional to be able to focus on the existing hair without continuing to be burdened with NEW hair growth. In order to achieve results and allow the patient to have some relief in shaving, I find it imperative that the patient begin to apply Vaniqa® in unison with the start of laser or IPL treatments. The Vaniqa® slows down the regrowth (which can be quite quick in biologically male patients) after each laser or IPL treatment. The entire laser or IPL treatment process can take months or even years to complete. By using the Vaniqa®, the patient experiences the feeling of "less hair" and a more feminine appearance much quicker. I can't imagine treating my transgender patients with only laser or IPL at this point. The combination of Vaniqa® and IPL has proven to be excessively more rewarding for the patient.

Again, this information is relevant because it outlines the struggles that patients with GD go through. Unfortunately, at the end of their struggles they are still left with unwanted hair (mainly on the face) that inhibits their complete transformation.

CHAPTER 13

THE ROAD TO RECOVERY

"We cannot change anything until we accept it.
Condemnation does not liberate, it oppresses."
—Carl Gustav Jung

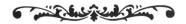

I have one phrase for you—**FAD!**

FACE IT

    ACCEPT IT

        DO SOMETHING ABOUT IT!

Before you can change anything in your life, you must first face your problem or situation and then admit there is a problem in the first place. Ignoring it, covering it up, and not talking about it will only compound the problem and cause even MORE problems.

The second step for me was to *truly* accept it. Not just pretend it is was "not a big deal," but honestly and completely accept the fact that I was a hairy person. The hair is a part of you and who you are, and that is just the way it is—like it or not. It won't go away if you avoid it. You don't have to live with it the rest of your life, but you do have to accept the fact that it is there and you have a problem. Even though I am pretty hair-free at this point, I still consider myself a "HAIRY" person. You could even possibly have a medical condition that needs attention. Once you accept it, you can fight it and do something about it!

I believe this book will teach you that you are certainly NOT ALONE. I wish I had that luxury years ago . The book can help you with FAD as well, which will ultimately prompt you to get help. This may sound strange, but so many women are so embarrassed about it that they don't dare talk about it, let alone ask anyone for help— even their closest friends, family or doctor. Once you can face it and accept it, the embarrassment goes out the window and you can finally ask for help. Talk to your doctor. You need to know if you have a more serious, underlying disorder that is causing the hair to grow in the first place. You might have been avoiding an important diagnosis in your medical life because you didn't FAD!

IN SUMMARY:

- Realize that you are not alone.
- Face it.
- Accept it.
- Talk to your physician and determine whether you have a disorder that may require medical treatment. Getting a firm diagnosis can put questions such as "Why am I so hairy?" into perspective!
- Do tons of research. Learn about your condition or disorder. Be armed with knowledge (this book can help you do that). Learn about how and why hair grows. Also, ask friends, relatives, your doctors, etc., if they recommend a certain facility. Finally, check the BBB (Better Business Bureau) and other organizations regarding the facility you choose to go to (also see Chapter 14 for a checklist).
- Set your own realistic expectations.(See Chapter 14)
- Decide on the treatment plan (laser, IPL, Vaniqa®, electrolysis, combination therapy).
- Make the commitment.
- DO SOMETHING ABOUT IT! Set up your consultations, decide on a facility, and book the appointment!

CHAPTER 14

WINNING THE BATTLE AGAINST UNWANTED HAIR GROWTH:

LASER AND INTENSE PULSED LIGHT PERMANENT HAIR REDUCTION

"Our belief at the beginning of a doubtful
undertaking is the one thing that insures the
successful outcome of our venture."
—William James

L.A.S.E.R. = **L**ight **A**mplification by **S**timulated **E**mission of **R**adiation

Lasers remove hair by the use of intense light energy which is absorbed by the pigmented portions of the hair follicle, with resultant "selective" destruction of these light-absorbing structures.

As with electrolysis, if any germinal tissue remains viable following treatment, new hair may appear. Laser is only effective in the active growth phase (anagen). If the hair is in the resting (telogen) stage of growth, there may be enough distance between the germinal tissue and the light-sensitive follicular structures that the germinal tissue is not harmed by the laser treatment and hair regrowth may occur. Laser treatments must typically be performed three to six times (and more in some cases) to obtain a permanent reduction in growth.

Laser hair removal is regulated by the U.S. Food and Drug Administration (FDA) and must be performed by certified professional personnel. Benefits of laser removal include the removal of many hairs in one session and only minor discomfort. Laser is most effective on dark hair, which absorbs more light energy in contrast to surrounding (lighter) tissue, an advantage in treatment of darker, terminal hair. Laser use is sometimes limited on lighter, colored hair, such as blond or red, and may result in reduced response to treatment. This can be a significant limitation of laser treatment.

> **KEY POINT: Laser is effective on dark hairsand is only effective on hairs in an active growthphase (anagen).**

The typical candidate for laser hair removal is Fitzpatrick Skin Type I, II, or III (see table 1 below). The use of intense pulsed light (IPL) or laser to selectively destroy follicular tissue poses some risk of unwanted heat transfer to surrounding tissue for all shades of complexion, particularly patients with dark skin (Fitzpatrick Skin Types IV-VI). To minimize this possibility, rapid advancements in laser technology tend toward longer wavelengths, shorter pulse duration, and cooling devices to be used in conjunction with laser therapy. These refinements have allowed laser technology to be safely used in people of darker skin color (Fitzpatrick Skin Types IV-VI) with less risk of blistering and pigment change (IPL is a great option). However, caution must still be employed when treating darker-skinned individuals.

Table 1. Fitzpatrick Skin Types

SKIN TYPE	DESCRIPTION
Type I	Very White or Freckled—always burns
Type II	White—usually burns
Type III	White to Olive—sometimes burns
Type IV	Brown—rarely burns
Type V	Dark Brown—very rarely burns
Type VI	Black—never burns

FITZPATRICK SKIN TEST --Skin Type Evaluation

"Genetic Disposition"

Question	0	1	2	3	4	Score
What is your natural eye color?	Light (*Blue, Gray or Green*)	Medium (*Blue, Gray or Green*)	Blue	Dark Brown	Brownish Black	
What is the natural color of your hair?	Sandy or Red	Blond	Chestnut or Dark Blond	Dark Brown	Black	
What is the color of your **NONEXPOSED** skin?	Reddish	Very Pale	Pale with Beige Tint	Light Brown	Dark Brown	
Do you have freckles on your **NON-EXPOSED** skin?	Many	Several	Few	Incidental	None	

Score_____

"Sun Reaction"

Question	0	1	2	3	4	Score
What happens if you stay in the sun too long?	Painful, redness, blistering, peeling	Blistering followed by peeling	Burns, sometimes followed by peeling	Rarely burns	Never burns	
To what degree do you turn brown?	Hardly or not at all	Light color tan	Reasonable tan	Tan very easily	Turn dark brown quickly	
Do you turn brown within several hours after sun exposure?	Never	Seldom	Sometimes	Often	Always	
How does your FACE react to the sun?	Very Sensitive	Sensitive	Normal	Very resistant	Never had a problem	

Score_____

"Tanning Habits"

Question	0	1	2	3	4	SCORE
When did you last expose the area TO BE TREATED to sun, tanning booth, cream or spray tan?	More than 3 months ago	2-3 months ago	1-2 months ago	Less than 1 month ago	Less than 2 weeks ago	
Did you expose the area to be treated to the sun?	Never	Hardly ever	Sometimes	Often	Always	

Score _____

TOTAL SCORE (Add all three totals above) _____

If your score is:	Then your FITZPATRICK skin type is:
0–7	I
8–16	II
17–24	III
25–30	IV
Over 30	V–VI

Note that while advancements in laser technology have made laser hair removal safer for dark-skinned people, laser should not be used on tanned skin. Tanning alters skin pigment and allows greater absorption of laser energy by the skin surrounding the hair follicle.

Some swelling and redness may result following laser treatment, but this usually subsides within 10 days of treatment (see Chapter 14 for details). Typically, hair does not fall out at the time of treatment. It may take up to two weeks for hair to fall out after follicular destruction. I call this the "Push-out Phase".

Other disadvantages of laser removal include the possibility of scarring; the inability to use on pigmented structures such as moles, freckles or keratosis; and the expense of treatment. *However, IPL machines CAN work on freckles and some other pigmented structures.

KEYPOINT: Lasers are capable of destroying the germinal tissue deep within a hair follicle by a process known as selective photothermolysis. The laser uses a particular wavelength and pulse duration of light to target a particular chromophore (colored object). The chromophore absorbs heat from the laser light and is destroyed, leaving surrounding tissue undamaged. Melanin is the primary chromophore for laser hair removal. Melanin is present in hair and skin. The darker the hair is, the greater the selectivity for the laser light. A color contrast between the skin and hair is necessary for selective hair removal without skin damage.

Types of Lasers

Laser hair removal was first approved by the FDA for Q-switched Neodymium: Yttrium-Aluminum-Garnet (Nd:YAG) (1064 nm, Soft Light system, ThermoLase Corp., San Diego, CA) laser in the late 1990s. These lasers used a carbon-mineral oil suspension to penetrate the hair follicle and act as an energy-absorbing chromophore. Carbon-mineral oil suspension did not provide a sufficient degree of selectivity, and is no longer used. However, long-pulsed Nd:YAG lasers which target melanin have been developed and are very effective and safe for use in darker-skinned individuals (see Chapter 15).

Long-pulse ruby lasers (694 nm, EpiLaser, Palomar Technologies, Lexington, MA, and EpiTouch, Sharplan Laser, Allendale, NJ) use the principle of selective thermolysis in which melanin is the target chromophore. Ruby lasers are not extensively used for hair removal anymore.

Long-pulse alexandrite lasers (755nm, PhotoGenica LPIR, Cynosure Inc., Chelmsford, MA) use thermokinetic selectivity to target melanin in the hair follicle. This allows the epidermis to cool more efficiently, thus reducing unwanted heat transfer to surrounding tissue. Long-pulse alexandrite lasers can be used safely on all skin types.

The LightSheer (Lumenis) is a diode laser operating at 810 nm with longer pulse durations (up to 30 milliseconds). Use of solid-state diode circuitry eliminates the need for a laser tube and reduces the size of the laser. Several studies have demonstrated long-pulsed diode lasers to be safe and effective for use in all skin types.

Supplier	Device Name
Long Pulse Nd: YAG 1064 nm	
Altus Medical	*CoolGlide*
	CoolGlide Excel
	Vantage
ICN US Photonics	*Varia*
Nd: YAG 1064 nm	
Candela	*GentleYAG*
Laserscope	*Lyra*
Focus Medical	*Lorad*
Continuum	*MedLite IV*
PhotoDerm/ ESC	*Vasculite Plus*
Cynosure	*SmartEpil II*
Depilase	*YAG LASE PLUS*
	TWIN YAG (1064 + 532)
Fotona	*Dualis VP (1065 + 532)*
	Dualis XP
Quantel Medical	*Athos*
Sciton	*Profile*
Telsar	*Softlight*
WaveLight	*Mydon*
Alexandrite 755nm	
Candela	*GentleLASE Plus*
	GentleLASE Limited Edition
Cynosure	*Apogee 6200*
	Apogee 9300
Depilase	*TWIN LASE (755 + 1065)*
Light Age	*EpiCare LP*
	EpiCare LP C
	EpiCare 2H
	EpiCare 4H
WaveLight	*Arion*
Diode 810 nm	
Asclepion- Meditec	*MeDioStar HC*
	MeDioStar C
Cynosure	*Apogee 100*
Dornier	*Medilas SkinPUlse S*
Iridex	*Apex 800*
Lumenis	*LightSheer ET*
	LightSheer ST
	LightSheer XC
Nidek	*EpiStar*
Opus	*F1 Diode Laser*
Palomar	*Palomar SLP1000*
Ruby 694 nm	
Asclepion-Meditec	*Ruby Star*

IPL: Intense Pulsed Light

A non-laser technology, Intense Pulsed Light (IPL)—or optically filtered xenon flashlamps—uses filters to select operating wavelengths of light (cut off at 690 nm) which allow light above this wavelength to pass through and affect hair. These systems are still being utilized with good results. However, at this point in time, IPL machines are classified as "lasers" and must follow appropriate laser protocols.

> **KEYPOINT:** Laser and IPL treatments cannot offer 100 percent hair removal. The proper term is actually "permanent hair reduction." There is a good chance that dormant follicles may grow hair months or even years after your treatment course. *Also, you may be left with fine, light hair. Therefore, the result would be "REDUCTION" as opposed to "REMOVAL" (See "Realistic Expectations" below for more details).

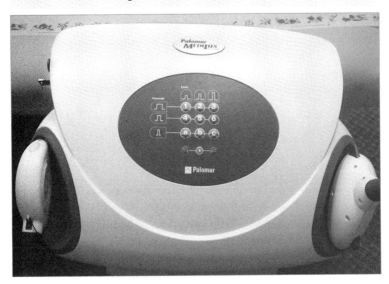

This is a picture of the machine I work with at my medical spa – the Palomar MediLux.

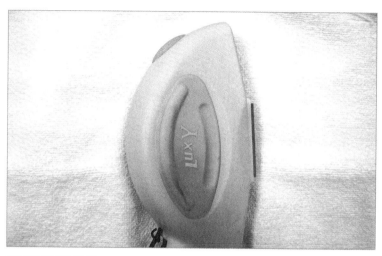

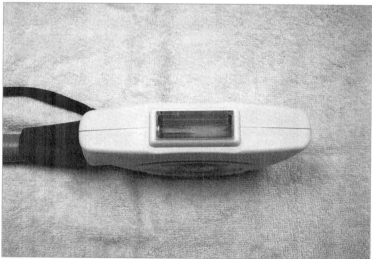

These are pictures of one of the actual handpieces that I work with. The spot size is 16 x 46-mm and is used on Fitzpatrick skin types I-IV. This handpiece is most commonly used in my facility, however, I cannot treat dark or tan skin with this one. The rectangle portion is placed directly on the skin (area to be treated).

As you can see, a large area is treated at one time.

This is one of the great benefits of IPL!

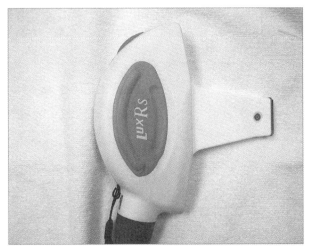

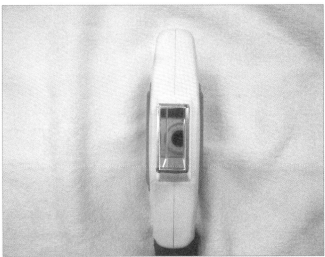

These are pictures of another handpiece that I work with. The spot size is 12 x 28-mm and is used on Fitzpatrick skin types I-IV (ALL SKIN TYPES). This is the handpiece that I treat darker skin and tan skin (although extremely tan, sunburned or recently tan skin is not recommended). The rectangle portion is placed directly on the skin (area to be treated). This handpiece has a higher spectral and fluence range. This allows patients with DARKER skin to receive hair reduction treatments. Yet another great benefit of IPL!

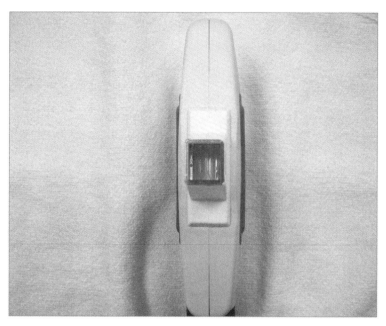

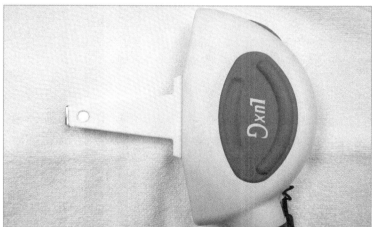

This is a picture of the final handpiece that I work with. The spot size is 12 x 12-mm and is used on Fitzpatrick skin types I-IV for pigmented and facial vascular lesions, including freckles. The treatment is called "Photofacial". I have personally obtained amazing results from the Photofacial treatments. However, results will vary for all people and once you achieve results, you must continue maintenance on your skin (as well as use a daily, full spectrum sunblock).

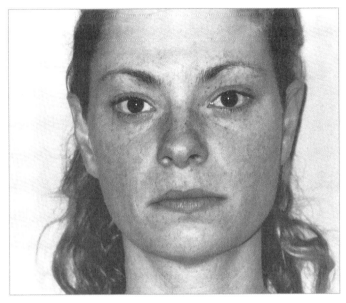

This is my "BEFORE" picture. It was taken in October 2004 before I started any treatments on my skin.

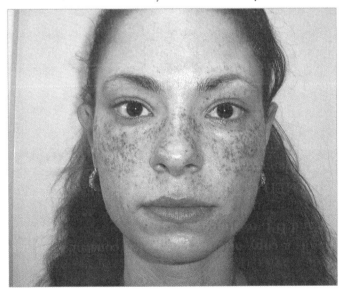

This picture was taken In November 2004 approximately 15 minutes after a high level Photofacial treatment.

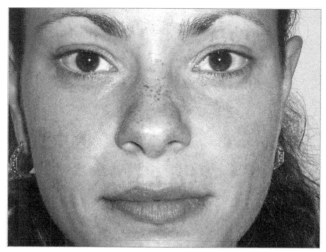

This picture was taken 10 days after the above Photofacial treatment. You can see the obvious results. The intense light attached to the darker pigment in my skin (basically freckles) and they got darker for a few days and then faded, almost completely.

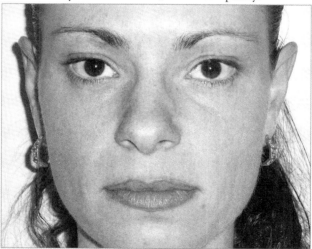

This picture was taken to show the long term results. It was taken in October 2005 after three photofacial treatments. Again, you can see the obvious results. The tone and texture of my skin overall improved drastically and my skin was more even. *These results were also achieved by obtaining numerous types of treatments and using specific products to help even the skin tone and maintain results. For questions – please email me at divinelaser@hotmail.com!

The Palomar MediLux System (the system that I work with) is designed to deliver light pulses (10-100ms) of broadband incoherent light to the predetermined target site.

The Palomar System indications for use are based upon the selective absorption of the emitted light by natural chromophores, including melanin and hemoglobin. The MediLux System is designed to effectively remove hair, benign pigmented lesions (e.g., solar lentigines—also known as age or liver spots and freckles) and actinic bronzing, and vascular lesions (e.g., telangiectasia, rosacea, spider veins, port-wine stain, flushing, etc.). For hair removal and treatment of pigmented lesions, the melanin in hair follicles and in hyper-pigmented basal layer cells is targeted by selecting the desired fluence with preset pulse width. Hemoglobin in the abnormal vasculature is the primary target in treatment of vascular lesions.

Treatment Intervals: Many laser/IPL clinics will give you the following generic treatment intervals:
- FACE/NECK: 3-4 Weeks
- UPPER BODY (shoulders to bikini area): 6-8 weeks
- LOWER BODY (bikini area and below): 8-10 weeks

> **KEYPOINT: *Since all humans are unique, everyone's growth-cycle intervals are unique as well and can vary significantly. This is very important to helping patients obtain treatments at proper intervals.**

Helpful Hint: Since hair follicles can only be permanently destroyed during the anagen (growth) phase, it can be beneficial to "try" to watch for what appears to be your specific NEW GROWTH CYCLE instead of booking treatments based on the above timescale.

After each laser/IPL treatment, you need to allow some time for the treated hairs to *push out*. This can look like new growth, but it is not. It can happen just a few days after a treatment, or it can take a few weeks. I give my patients another timescale to work with: three weeks for face, five weeks for upper body, and seven weeks for lower body. I call this the *push out phase*. Although you can shave during the *push out phase*, I advise patients to note the end of their phase (if they are treated on their chin on the 1st of the month, the end of their *push out phase* would be the 21st) and shave on that day (the 21st in this scenario). Then, when they start to see hair growth after this point, it can possibly be a NEW GROWTH CYCLE. You should make your next appointment within 14 days of seeing the new growth.*This is certainly not a guarantee, but I feel it is better than blindly making appointments and hoping to catch a NEW GROWTH CYCLE.

I have had pretty good results using these theories. However, sometimes this is difficult to maintain, and patients make their appointments based on average intervals. If so, patients should reschedule their appointment if they have NO growth at all by their appointment date. If there is no growth at all, that would be a waste of a treatment altogether. *However *(sorry to complicate this further)*, if the growth gets too long (meaning the actual length of the hairs are very long) by the appointment date, you probably missed your NEW GROWTH CYCLE! You want to get a treatment as soon as you see the hairs 'pop.'

I know this sounds extremely complicated, but you are investing a lot of time and money into your treatments. Anything you can do to improve results is worth the extra effort. Good providers will help you work through this and will do their best to treat you appropriately.

> **KEYPOINT: Before you begin treatments, the amount of hair you see above the skin is not necessarily 100 percent of all the hairs that you truly have. Due to the different cycles of hair growth (anagen, telogen and**

catagen), you may only physically see about 50 to 60 percent of the total amount of hairs. Once you start laser/IPL treatments, the hairs are sometimes prompted to start growing more in unison. As you progress with treatments and kill some of the hairs in the anagen phase, your cycles may start to shift, and instead of only 50 percent of your hairs being visible above the skin, now 75 percent is above the skin. We may have killed off 20 percent, but in reality, after a few treatments you may now see 55 percent of your total amount of hairs above the skin. This would appear to be MORE than what you had when you started, but in actuality, it is not. I call this MASSIVE PUSH OUT.

Realistic Expectations

Expectations of Systemic and Medicinal Treatment

The treatment of hirsutism requires patience because hair follicles have a life cycle of about six months. Most medications must be taken for three to six months before a noticeable improvement occurs. In the meantime, the existing hair can be mechanically removed or bleached, and some women may continue to use these methods in combination with medication. Your doctor will monitor the progress of treatment and may repeat any tests if he or she is concerned about an underlying condition. If a medication is ineffective initially, your doctor may change the dose or recommend a trial of a different medication. It is important to have realistic goals for the reduction of body hair and to place these goals within the context of your racial and ethnic background.

Expectations of Laser/IPL Treatments

In my practice, I make sure that "realistic expectations" are clearly explained to all of my patients. As a patient, you should also have your own expectations as well. You are paying for a service, but you are also signing up to take part in a treatment plan. You must be committed to follow the recommended rules and guidelines and understand the realistic results and side affects. You must voluntarily take part in this program. Nothing in life is guaranteed, and that is true in this case as well. I can, however, tell you that IPL/laser treatments offer great results, but, it works differently and at different levels for each person. You must go into this knowing that what works for one person may not work the *exact* same for you. Don't expect miracles; that way you will not be disappointed. Most of my patients initially book a consultation with the expectation that they will become 100 percent hair-free forever. I quickly let them know that this is completely unrealistic and clinically impossible.

KEYPOINT: You are born with a predetermined number of hair follicles. You have dormant follicles and active follicles. Only active follicles (anagen phase) can be destroyed. Dormant follicles can and probably will grow hair at some point down the road. *Treated areas will be smooth but will likely have some sporadic growth even after the full treatment process is completed. Touch-up treatments are very common.

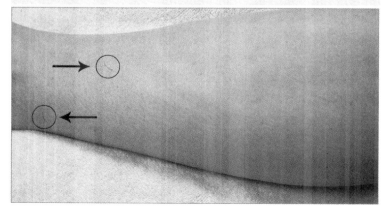

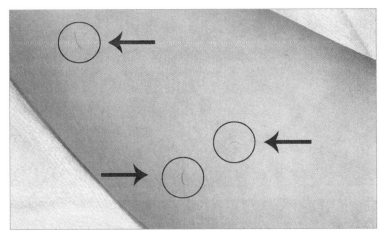

These are pictures of my long-term results of laser and IPL treatments on my lower leg. It was taken on March 18, 2006. I have had a total of 11 treatments of a mix of laser *(Candela)* and IPL *(Palomar MediLux)* treatments by this point. I started treatments over 3 years ago, and my last "touch-up" treatment was in September 2005. I have not shaved my legs in over two years. I am left with a very minimal number of hairs (you can actually count them in this picture). Hopefully this photo can help you visualize what the "END RESULT" of laser/IPL treatments can look like *(of course my results and your results will not be exactly the same).* My legs are not 100 percent hair-free, but I am completely satisfied with the smoothness of my legs because I had **REALISTIC EXPECTATIONS**.

Patient and Provider Expectations and Responsibilities

Over the past 18 years, I have been on both ends of the spectrum. I have been both a patient and a provider. I have learned a lot from both perspectives and I firmly believe that we (as patients) need to take responsibility for our decisions and actions. On the other hand, I also firmly believe that we (as

Laura M. Regan

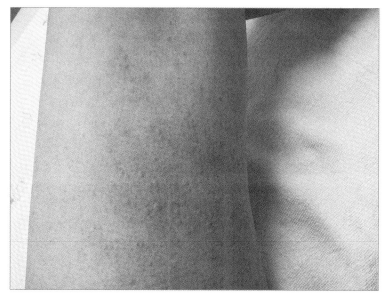

This picture was taken of a leg about ten minutes after a high level IPL hair reduction treatment. This is a great picture of what epidermal erythema (redness) and follicular edema (bumps) look like after a treatment. The area returned to normal within 24 hours.
*Keep in mind – results vary person to person. This is just a visual for you so you understand what "might" happen.

professionals) also need to take responsibility for our work as well as educating our patients to the best of our ability. Part of the responsibility of a provider is to continue our education within our field of expertise. It is our *responsibility* to keep up-to-date on new and changing methods of treatment, technological advancements, disorder updates, etc. Providers also need to be in tune with their patients from a demographic and "human" standpoint. We should understand and be sympathetic to our patients' individual concerns, lifestyles, disorders, goals of treatment, and the psychological impact that hirsutism has on them.

KEYPOINT: Patient and provider responsibilities are essential components needed to achieve effective results in a safe and comfortable environment.

You (the patient) must:

- Be honest up front about the true severity of your disorder and all areas that grow hair.

- Be honest about your medical history and all issues involved (especially those that can be contraindications). This is in your best interest and is for your safety as well.

- Be completely ready for the entire process and be committed and prepared to stick with the treatments.

- Be educated and armed with knowledge about the disorders involved; risks; how treatments work; tips and helpful hints; why and how the hair grows, etc.

- Be a "patient" patient—results don't happen overnight.

- Persevere.

- Have realistic expectations. Set your goals up front and share them with your provider to see if they are realistic and attainable.

- Follow all pre- and post-care instructions closely.

I also believe that we (as professionals)—physicians (including OBGYNs), RNs, laser/IPL technicians, and all other providers—can help by:

- Adding "Unwanted Facial Hair" to the patient history forms and initiating the discussion on the topic (many patients are so embarrassed by the condition that they won't start the conversation. By adding "Hirsutism" to their paperwork, we can help gently initiate the conversation).

- Letting patients know that there are options and solutions.
- Letting patients know that they are not alone.
- Realizing that we (as the providers) may not be able to physically "see" the patients' unwanted hair growth by just looking at them.
- Being compassionate.
- Being honest and explaining "realistic expectations" of the end result (don't promise too much!).
- Explaining the commitment that is involved and required.
- Educating patients and keeping them informed.
- Continuing our education in all aspects of our field.

You have learned in the earlier paragraphs just how laser and IPL physically work. With that said, you also know that the end result is actually permanent hair *reduction,* not permanent hair *removal* (if a provider promises permanent removal, go somewhere else!). A viable "realistic expectation" is to significantly reduce the hair growth slowly over time. By the end of your treatment plan, you should expect to have smoother skin in the area (or areas), provided that you follow all pre- and post-care instructions as well as commit to and continue with treatments as advised.

Contraindications and Alternatives

Unfortunately, there are some people who will not be able to receive laser treatments. I have done enough research over the years to find alternative treatments or options to a few of these contraindications. Obviously, patients will not receive the same results that lasers or IPL can offer, but it is important to be aware of all your options. My point is, don't give up! If being "hairy" is a significant problem for you, understand and research your options. I have worked with many patients who were not candidates for laser or IPL. Initially they were very disappointed and were ready to give up. I made the effort to educate them and give them very honest and REALISTIC expectations. In most cases, even slightly reducing or slowing down regrowth made a world of difference. It takes patience, commitment, perseverance, education and realistic expectations (you should be getting pretty familiar with these words at this point!).

Contraindications to IPL treatment include but are not limited to:

1) Pregnancy/Breast-Feeding
ALTERNATIVE : NONE. In my opinion, just wait it out! It is not worth the risk. Get yourself good and hairy! Let your hormones rage, then give birth, then start your treatments!

2) Diabetes
ALTERNATIVE: Vaniqa®. (See Chapter 19 or consult with your physician).

3) Seizures
ALTERNATIVE: Consult with your physician (Vaniqa® might be a good option).

4) Gold Therapy
Taking, or ever having taken Gold Therapy *(actually called "Gold Salts,"—not the 24-karat variety—Gold Therapy was originally developed as a treatment for tuberculosis; although it was ineffective for TB, gold soon proved its worth against inflammatory arthritis).*
ALTERNATIVE: NONE other than Vaniqa®.

5) Taking Accutane
ALTERNATIVE: Consult your physician OR wait at least one full year after last dose to start treatments (you can use Vaniqa® in the interim).

6) Antivirals (Antibiotics)**MOST COMMON**

ALTERNATIVE: You must wait 8 to 12 weeks after last dose (depending on the type of antibiotic and the laser technicians' requirements). *Also see below list of drugs that cause photo-sensitivity.

7) True Red Hair

ALTERNATIVE: Meladine™ and/or Vaniqa® (see Chapters 18 and 19).

8) Blond, Gray, White Hair

ALTERNATIVE: Meladine™ and/or Vaniqa® (see Chapters 18 and 19).

9) CERTAIN DRUGS THAT MAY CAUSE PHOTO-SENSITIVITY:

There are many drugs that can cause photosensitivity *(an abnormally heightened response, especially of the skin, to sunlight or ultraviolet radiation, caused by certain disorders or chemicals and characterized by a toxic or allergic reaction).*

ALTERNATIVE: If you are taking any of these medications, consult with the laser or IPL professional for your alternatives. Not all of the medications listed below completely inhibit you from receiving treatments. Some drugs may just cause minor photosensitivity, and you can continue with treatments. On the other hand, some drugs cause intense sensitivity; you may need to wait a determined amount of time before resuming treatments. It is also your decision to stop medications in order to receive treatments. Consult your physician.

The following is a list of medications that may cause photosensitivity.

THE LIST PROVIDED MAY NOT INCLUDE ALL MEDICATIONS

ACNE MEDICATIONS	**ANTIHISTAMINES AND ANTIPSYCHOTICS**	**HERBAL/ORGANIC**
Tretinoin (Retin-A)	Astemizole (Hismanal)	
Azithromycin (Zithromax)	Chlorpromazinc (Thorazinc; and others)	St. John's Wort
Accutane	Cyprohepatadine (Periactin)	
Demaclocycline (Declomycin; and others)	Fluphenazine (Permitil; Prolixin)	
Doxycycline (Vibramycin; and others)	Diphenhydramine (Benadryl)	**HORMONAL**
ANTICANCER DRUGS	Haloperidol (Haldol)	All birth control drugs (oral
Griseofulvin (fulvicin-U/F; and others)	Loratadine (Claritin)	contraceptives)
Dacarbazine (DTIC-Dome)	Perphenazine (Trilafon)	All hormonal drugs
Methacycline (rondomycin)	Terfenadine (Seldene)	
Fluorouracil (Fluoroplex; others)	Piperacetazine (Quide)	**HYPOGLYCEMICS**
Nalidixic acid (NegGram; and others)	Prochlorperazine (Compazine; and others)	Acetohexamide (Dymelor)
Methotrexate (Mexate; others)	**ANTI-INFLAMMATORY DRUGS (NSAIDs)**	Chlorpropamide (Diabinese; Insulase)
OxyteWacyclines (Terramycin; and others)	Promethazine (Phenergan; and others)	Glipizide (Glucotrol)
Procarbazine (Matulane, Natulan)Sulfacyntine (Renoquid)	All nonsteroidal anti-inflammatory drugs e.g.	Glyburide (Diabeta, Micronase)
Vinblastine (Veiban)	Thioridazine Hydrochloride, Mellaril	Tolazamide (Tolinase)
Sulfamethazine (Neotrizine; and others)	Hydrochloride	Tolbutamide (Orinase; and others)
Sulfamethizoic (Thiosulfil; and others)	Ibuprofen (Motrin)	
ANTIDEPRESSANTS	Trifluperazine (Stelazine; and others)	**SUNCREENS**
Sulfamethoxazole (Gantanol; and others)	Naprosen	Benzophenones (Aramis, Clinique, etc.)
Amitriptyline (Elavil; others)	Triflupromazine (Vesprin)	Cinnamates (Aramis, Estee Lauder, etc.)
Sulfamethoxazolc-trimethoprim (BacU'im; Septra)	Naproxen (Anaprox, Naprosyn)	Dioxybenzone (Solbar Plus, etc.)
Clomipramine (Anafranil)	Trimeprazine (Termaril)	Oxybenzone (Eclipse, PreSun, Shade, etc.)
Sulfasalazinc (Azulfidine; and others)	Orudis, Feldene, Voltaren, etc.	PABA (PreSun, etc.)
Desipramine (Norpramin; Petroiliam)	Etodolac (Lodine)	PABA esters (Block Out, Sea & Ski, Eclipse, etc.)
Sulfathiazolc	**ANTIMICROBIALS/ANTIBIOTIC**	
Doxepin (Adapin; Sinequan)	Azithromycin (Zithromax)	**MISCELLANEOUS**
Sulfisoxazole (Gantrisin; and others)	Demaclocycline (Declomycin; and others)	Benzocaine
Imipramine (Tofranil; and others)	Doxycycline (Vibramycin; and others)	Carbamazepine (Tegretol)
Tetracyclines (Achromysin; minocin)	Griseofulvin (fulvicin-U/F; and others	Coal Tar, e.g. Tegrin, Zetar, etc.
Isocarboxazid (Marplan)	Methacycline (rondomycin)	Oral estazolam (ProSom)
	Nalidixic acid (NegGram; and others)	Etretinate (Tegison)
	OxyteWacyclines (Terramycin; and others)	Felbamate (Felbatol)
	Sulfacyntine (Renoquid)	Gabapentin (Neurontin)
	Sulfamethazine (Neotrizine; and others)	Gold salts (Myochrysine, Ridaura,
	Sulfamethizoic (Thiosulfil; and others)	
	Sulfamethoxazole (Gantanol; and others)	

Maprotiline (Ludiomil)	Sulfamethoxazolc-trimethoprim (BacU'im; Septra)	Solganol)
ANTIPARASITICS	Sulfasalazinc (Azulfidine; and others)	Hexachlorophene (pHisoHex, etc.)
Notriptylin (Aventyl; Pamelor)	Sulfathiazolc	isotretinoin (Accutane)
Bithionol (Bitin)	Sulfisoxazole (Gantrisin; and others	
Protriptyline (Vivactil)	Tetracyclines (Achromysin; minocin)	
Chloroquine (Aralen)	**DIURETICS**	**PERFUME OILS**
Sertraline (Zoloft)	Nabumetone (Ralafen)	
Mefloquine (Lariam)	Acetazolamide (Diamox)	Sandalwood, cedar, musk, etc.
Trimipramine (Surmontil)	Oxaprozine (Daypro)	quinidine sulfate & gluconate
Pyrvinium pamoate (Povan, Vanquin)	Amiloride (Midamor)	selegiline (Deprenyl, Eldepryl)
Venlafaxine (Effexor)	Bendroflumethiazide (Naturetin; and others)	tretinoin (Retin-A, Vitamin A Acid)
Quinine		zolpidem (Ambien)

167

KEYPOINT: Your doctor or laser/IPL professional will make the final determination if you are on one of the listed medications. *If you are taking any other medication on a regular basis that is NOT on the list, it is wise to check with your physician, pharmacist and/or laser/IPL professional to make sure it does not cause photosensitivity.

Pre- and Post-Care Instructions

It is important to closely follow PRE- and POST-CARE INSTRUCTIONS. By doing so, you can significantly decrease side effects and risks.

KEYPOINT: Strict conformity to all instructions can help you obtain SAFE and more effective results.

Below is the actual form that I give to all of my patients:

Pre-Care Instructions:

1) Refrain from ingesting caffeine of any kind (it can make you more sensitive to pain).
2) Avoid sun exposure (tanning), tanning beds or sprays as well as self-tanning lotions for four to eight weeks prior to each treatment. This can help reduce the chance of dark or light spots (hypo- or hyperpigmentation).
3) Refrain from tweezing, waxing, sugaring, electrolysis or other depilatory methods for at least four weeks prior to treatment (and for the duration course).
4) Cleanly (but gently) shave area to be treated (use hair conditioner to help avoid razor burn).
5) Moisturize skin on a daily basis. Healthy, hydrated skin will handle the treatments much better.

Post-Treatment Instructions:

1) Immediately after the treatments, there should be

redness and bumps at the treatment area, which may last up to two hours or up to several days in some cases. It is normal for the treated area to feel like sunburn for a few hours. You should use a cold compress if needed. If any crusting, apply an antibiotic cream. Some physicians recommend aloe vera gel or some other after-sunburn treatment such as Desitin, CU3 or Aquaphor. Darker-pigmented people may have more discomfort than lighter-skinned people and may require the aloe vera gel or an antibiotic ointment longer.

What is CU3? Complex CU3 is an intensive repair crème and post-laser lotion. CU3 is made by ProCyte Corporation (see resources).

2) Makeup may be used after the treatment, unless there is epidermal blistering. It is recommended to use new makeup to reduce the possibility of an infection. Just make sure that you have moisturizer on under your makeup. In fact, moisturizer will help the dead hair exfoliate from the follicle, so use moisturizer frequently and freely on the treated area. Any moisturizer without alpha-hydroxy acids will work.

3) Avoid sun exposure to reduce the chance of dark or light spots for two months. Use Sunscreen SPF 25 or higher at all times throughout the treatment. Also avoid tanning beds and tanning creams for at least four to six weeks.

4) Avoid picking or scratching the treated skin.

5) Refrain from tweezing, waxing, sugaring, electrolysis or other depilatory methods in-between treatments and for the entire duration course of treatments, as it will prevent you from achieving your best results. *Remember—shaving is acceptable and even recommended!

6) If you shower quickly after the laser treatments and use soap, deodorant, etc., the treated area should be washed gently with a mild soap. Skin should be patted dry and NOT rubbed. You may apply deodorant after 24 hours.

7) Anywhere from 5 to 30 days after the treatment, shedding of the hair may occur (the "PUSH-OUT PHASE), and this may appear as new hair growth. This is not new hair growth, but dead hair pushing its way out of the follicle. You can help the hair exfoliate by washing or wiping with a washcloth (wait a few days after treatment for the skin to heal). You can also use a lint roll believe it or not, and roll away some of the dead hairs! This can help avoid in-grown hairs as well.

8) Hair regrowth occurs at different rates on different areas of the body. New hair growth will not occur for at least three weeks after the treatment.

9) Please note: Stubble, representing dead hair being shed from the hair follicle, will appear within 10 to 30 days from the treatment date. This is normal, and they may fall out quickly. You can use a lint roll to help move along the hairs.

Side Affects And Risks

Below is the actual form that I give to all of my patients:

1) However slight, there is a risk of scarring.

2) Short-term effects may include reddening (Epidermal Erythema), mild burning, small bumps (Follicular Edema), temporary bruising or blistering. Hyperpigmentation (browning) and hypo-pigmentation (lighting) have also been noted after treatment. These conditions usually resolve within three to six

months, but permanent color change is a rare risk. Avoiding sun exposure before and after the treatment reduces the risk of color change.

3) Infection: Although infection following treatment is unusual, bacterial, fungal and viral infections can occur. Herpes simplex virus infections around the mouth can occur following a treatment. This applies to individuals with no known history of herpes simplex virus infections in the mouth area. Should any type of skin infection occur, additional treatments or medical antibiotics may be necessary.

4) Bleeding: Pinpoint bleeding is rare, but can occur following treatment procedures. Should bleeding occur, additional treatment may be necessary.

5) Allergic Reactions: In rare cases, local allergies to tape, preservatives used in cosmetics or topical preparations and post-laser lotions have been reported. Systemic reactions (which are more serious) may result in prescription medicines.

6) Exposure of eyes to the light could harm your vision. You must wear protective eyewear during treatments.

7) Compliance with the aftercare guidelines is crucial for healing, prevention of scarring, and hyperpigmentation.

8) Patients must disclose, in their best interest, all medical conditions and current medications, both prescription and over-the-counter, prior to treatment, as well as any changes before subsequent treatments.

9) Patients must disclose, in their best interest, recent exposure, whether direct or indirect, to sun or tanning lamps. Sun or tanning-lamp exposure and use of self-tanners may increase your chance of complications and hypo- and/or hyperpigmentation.

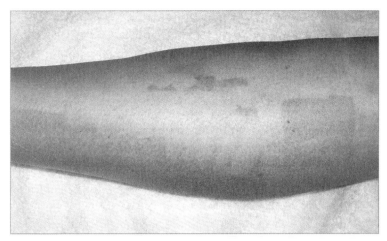

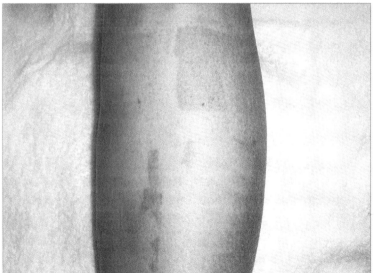

These pictures were taken in April 2006 of a patient who failed to tell her provider that she had recent sun exposure. The patient was too tan and should not have been treated. The end result is HYPO or HYPERPIGMEN-TATION (diminished or excessive pigmentation or coloring), and as you can see, it is quite serious. It took this patient over 6 months to even out the discoloration.

Steps to Take to Ease or Prevent Certain Side Effects

As I have stressed, it is important to understand that as a patient, it is your responsibility to be as educated about the laser or IPL process as possible *(see patient responsibilities in Chapter 14)*. You must follow pre- and post-care instructions as well to insure the best possible results and to also decrease the possibility of side effects. There are many things you can do as an educated, committed consumer to help ease or decrease the risks involved:

*The below is a bit repetitive but these guidelines are so important so I wanted to repeat them as much as possible!

- **BURNS:** To help lower the risks of burns you can:
  - ✓ Ask your provider to use ice packs or cold rollers during the treatment (or bring your own).
  - ✓ Apply cold compresses after the treatment (at home).
  - ✓ Avoid taking medications that cause photosensitivity.
  - ✓ Stay out of the sun a few days prior to and after treatments.
  - ✓ Avoid spray tans or sunless tanners a few weeks before treatment.
  - ✓ Come in with very clean skin (all makeup removed).
  - ✓ Apply Aquaphor, CU3, Aloe.
- **SCARRING:**
  - ✓ Follow the above guidelines for burns.
  - ✓ DO NOT PICK or irritate scabs or blisters if they occur.

- **PAIN LEVEL:**
  ✓ Avoid caffeine prior to treatment.
  ✓ Continue to apply ice packs at home.
  ✓ For "sunburn-like" pain after treatment, use ice packs, apply Aquaphor, 100 percent pure aloe vera gel (you can store this in the refrigerator to add cooling), and/or CU3 Intensive Repair Cream.
  ✓ Avoid treatment on or around your menstrual cycle (you are more sensitive to pain at this time)
  ✓ Recent sun exposure (not necessarily a burn) can cause more heat which causes more pain

What You Must Consent To

You will be asked to sign an *INFORMED CONSENT* form in order to proceed with treatments. Be sure to read the entire form and understand it completely.

Here is a copy of a recommended consent form used for laser and IPL treatments.

INFORMED CONSENT FOR HAIR REMOVAL
Customer's Name: _____**Date:** _____

Treatment sites: mono-brow, lip, chin, neck, face, arms, fingers, chest, areola, underarms, back, buttocks, bikini, labia, thighs, lower legs, feet and toes.
Combinations: _____
Previous hair removal methods _____
(shaving, tweezing, waxing, depilatories, electrolysis, laser)

The purpose of this procedure is to diminish or remove unwanted hair. The procedure requires more than one treatment and may produce permanent hair removal. The total number of treatments will vary between individuals. On occasion, there are patients that do not respond to treatments. The treated hair should exfoliate or push out in approximately 2-3 weeks.

Contraindications to IPL treatment include, but are not limited to: Being pregnant, diabetic, seizures, taking (or ever have taken) Gold Therapy, taking Accutane or Antivirals (Antibiotics). *If you are taking Accutane or Antibiotics, please advise the laser technician. You cannot receive treatment at this time.

Patient has disclosed all medical conditions and current medications, both prescription and over-the-counter prior to treatment, and any changes before subsequent treatments. I have been completely honest in divulging the above information as well as my exposure, whether direct or indirect, to sun or tanning lamps. Sun or tanning-lamp exposure may increase my chance of complications.

Alternative methods are waxing, shaving, electrolysis and chemical epilation.

The following are problems that may occur with the hair removal system.

1) However slight, **there is a risk of scarring**.

2) **Short-term effects may include reddening, mild burning, temporary bruising or blistering.** Hyperpigmentation (browning) and **hypo-pigmentation** (lighting) have also been noted after treatment. These conditions usually resolve within 3-6 months, but **permanent color change is a rare risk**. Avoiding sun exposure before and after the treatment reduces the risk of color change.

Infection: Although infection following treatment is unusual, bacterial, fungal and viral infections can occur. Herpes simplex virus infections around the mouth can occur following a treatment. This applies to individuals with no known history of herpes simplex virus infections in the mouth area. Should any type of skin infection occur, additional treatments or medical antibiotics may be necessary.

3) **Bleeding**: Pinpoint bleeding is rare, but can occur following treatment procedures. Should bleeding occur, additional treatment may be necessary.

4) **Allergic Reactions**: In rare cases, local allergies to tape, preservatives used in cosmetics or topical preparations have been reported. Systemic reactions (which are more serious) may result in prescription medicines.

5) I understand that exposure of my eyes to light could harm my vision. I must keep the eye protection goggles on at all times.

6) Compliance with the aftercare guidelines is crucial for healing, prevention of scarring, and hyperpigmentation.

7) Patient has disclosed all medical conditions and current medications, both prescription and over-the-counter, prior to treatment, and any changes before subsequent treatments. I have been completely honest in divulging the above information as well as my exposure, whether direct or indirect, to sun or tanning lamps. **Sun or tanning-lamp exposure may increase my chance of complications**.

8) Cancellation Policy: I understand that I will be charged for my full treatment total (or a full treatment will be deducted from total remaining package treatments) if I do not cancel my appointment at least 24 hours in advance (preferably 48 hours). Thank you for understanding.

9) I have received and carefully read a copy of pre-and post-care instructions for IPL treatments. I understand that not adhering to the pre- and post-care

instructions provided to me may increase my chance of complications.

Occasionally, unforeseen mechanical problems may occur and your appointment will need to be rescheduled. We will make every effort to notify you prior to your arrival at the office. Please be understanding if we cause you any inconvenience.

ACKNOWLEDGMENT:
My questions regarding the procedure have been answered satisfactorily. I understand the procedure and accept the risks. I hereby release _____ (individual) and _____ (facility) and _____ (doctor) from all liabilities associated with the above indicated procedure.

Client/Guardian Signature _____

Date _____

Laser Technician Signature _____

Date _____

Important Considerations When Choosing a Laser/IPL Provider

You are now armed with knowledge! This can help you achieve better, safer results, as well as help you avoid wasting your precious time and money!

Once you have determined that IPL/laser hair removal is right for you, it is time to make some important decisions. First, you must decide what kind of equipment is suited for your needs. The decision to start treatment will certainly change your life, so you must be serious about it from the very beginning.

Your body is sacred; you should do your homework before you let anyone "work" on you. You will get more out of your treatment if you educate yourself on how the equipment actually works. I have received treatments from numerous types of lasers, but I am most familiar with IPL (Intense Pulsed Light). I chose IPL for my business and have had amazing results.

It is also important to visit a few clinics and get some consultations before making your final decision as well. At this point, you have had a crash course in lasers and IPL. You are officially an educated consumer. Let your new knowledge guide you and help you reach your goal. The education you have obtained can make the difference between just getting some treatments, and getting real permanent results. Make one or two (or even more if you wish) consultation appointments (also see Chapter 11 for preteen and teenage patients). After your meetings, you will know which facility is right for you. Go with your instinct. It is important to feel comfortable with the technician and be confident in his or her abilities. Your gut will help you with this.

You are now ready to start treatment! Here is a checklist you can use. ***The items indicated in this list are just some of my personal recommendations. There could be many other important issues and factors to take into consideration based on personal issues, desires and requirements.**

- Are they a member of the Better Business Bureau? If so, are there any complaints filed against them.
- Is their equipment FDA approved?
- Do they have proper licensing per state (see resources in the back of the book)
- Ask for their credentials.
- What kind of machine do they use?

- Review their credentials
- What kind of experience and training do they have?
- Are their prices at least average?(Do a comparison between a few places. In Arizona, an average price for a chin treatment for example is $55-70.00 per treatment)
- Do they have testimonials you can review?
- Who is their medical director?
- Do they have continuing education for their staff and technicians?
- Did they honestly explain the treatment intervals to you?
- Are they able to work on dark skin (if applicable)? (see Chapter 15.)
- What kind of insurance do they have?
- Do they wear gloves and sanitize the equipment, bed etc.?
- Can you get a consultation? If so, is there a charge?
- Do they have options when it comes to blond, gray or white hair (if applicable)? (See Chapter 18 and 19.)
- Can you get a test spot?
- Do they work on young (preteen and teenage) patients (if applicable)? Are they educated about their disorders? (See Chapter 11.)
- Are they familiar with some of the disorders that can cause hair growth?
- Do they work on transgender patients (if applicable)? Are they educated about their special issues? (See Chapter 12.)
- Were they honest about how many treatments you will need? (Honesty is important.)
- Do they claim permanent hair REMOVAL? If so, go somewhere else!

- Did they clearly cover the true risks and side effects?
- Did they go over realistic expectations with you

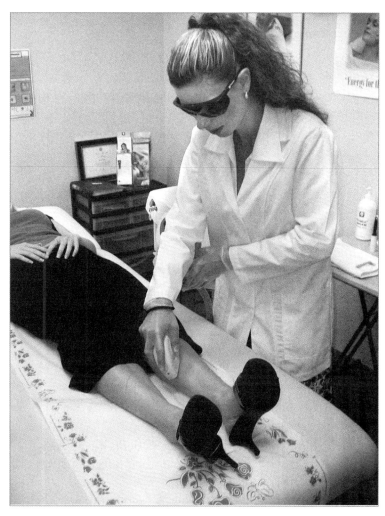

This is a picture of me working on a patients leg with the Palomar Medilux system (as you can see, both the patient and provider must wear protective goggles to protect their eyes from the intense light).

IPL Treatment Protocol

Many perspective patients ask questions like "What is involved in a treatment" or "What are treatments like?" In order to help answer these questions, I wrote a brief synopsis of what happens (and what should happen) during a typical IPL treatment. Please keep in mind that this information is from my own personal experience working with the Palomar Medilux system and may not be for everyone or apply to all situations. This is merely a brief description of what the provider and patient should do:

1) If you are a new, first time patient, you should get a thorough consultation. Just a few important items that should be covered are:
   • All paperwork should be signed and discussed thoroughly
   • Pre and post care instructions given and explained
   • Brief overview of why and how hair grows
   • Treatment intervals explained
   • Skin evaluation (Fitzpatrick Test)
   • Treatment protocol explained (how the machine actually works)
   • Realistic expectations discussed;
   • Test spot done (if necessary);
   • Pricing
   • Side-effects discussed
   *There is a lot more involved but this is a good start.

2) Ask client if they are on their period or if they had caffeine in the past 3 hours. If so, this can cause them to be more sensitive to "pain"
3 Ask client if they have started new medications (specifically antibiotics that cause photosensitivity) or have had recent sun exposure or used tanning sprays or lotions in the past week. If they answer yes, do not treat! Re-schedule for appropriate time.
4) A few nice touches would be to have some soft, spa music playing for relaxation and/or aromatherapy to calm and sooth
5) Have a stress ball on hand. Some patients like to squeeze the stress ball during the treatment

6) Prep area(s) to be treated:
- Look for makeup and/or lotion (all residue must be removed in order to avoid impeding the light to penetrate the area). Wipe down area(s) with alcohol and/or wet towels. You can also use Lux Lotion which is basically a sugar water (from Palomar).
- Shave area if necessary. Patients should be shaved prior to coming in but if they are not, many facilities charge extra to do it for them. *For small areas (like the face), use a TINKLE (a small razor usually used on eyebrows. You can find them on the internet or in pharmacy stores like CVS) . If you do have to shave for the patient, make sure to use a LINT ROLL to completely remove all loose hairs.

7) Offer a head and/or knee pillow for comfort

8) Protective Eyewear: both the patient and provider must protect their eyes. Providers can use a special pair of goggles from Palomar that automatically "blink" when each pulse goes off. Patients can use goggles, eye pillows or eye guards

9) Offer a mouth guard (or place a cotton pad between teeth and gums) for sensitive treatments like upper lip. The shock can go through the teeth and feel uncomfortable.

10) Numb the area(s): Some patients request or require numbing in order to be able to treat them effectively. If so, I use either PHOTO-CAINE (prescription medication) or ZCAINE (from Creative Technologies Inc.). You must be sure to thoroughly remove all residue before starting the treatment. Also use the creams strictly as prescribed.

11) Always let the patient know what is happening and what you are doing. They cannot see well through their goggles so you don't want to scare or shock them.

12) Mark the area(s) to be treated: If you are treating a large area like full legs, you will need to mark the area into sections so you do not miss spots. Since laser or IPL cannot see "Red"—you can use a red marker. However, this can be messy (especially if you use a cold

roller) so I recommend using a small towel as a guide

13) Have an index card handy. Since the hand piece is flat but some areas you treat will be curved (like the forehead), you must cover the area that the hand piece does not touch or else it can cause a burn. Index cards work the best for this.

14) Use gloves – always! I use latex-free because many people are allergic to latex.

15) Start the treatment! First cool the area with an ice pack or cold roller (see picture – you can order these from Palomar) and then place the hand piece directly onto the skin. Make sure you overlap in order to avoid missed spots. Cool down the hand piece with a cryogen spray after every 4-6 hits. I use "COOL SPRAY" from Palomar. Watch the skin for an instant major reaction. *Beware that some patients may not be 100% truthful about new medications they started or new sun exposure they had. This can cause an immediate reaction. If you see this, stop treatment immediately.

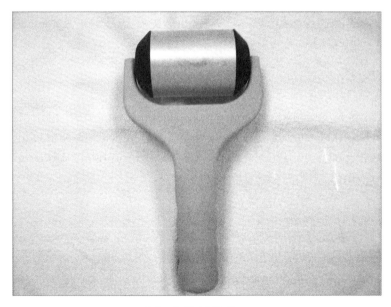

Metal Cold Roller

16) Apply ointments immediately after treatment:
- You can apply COMPLEX CU3 POST LASER LOTION or COMPLEX CU3 INTENSIVE TISSUE REPAIR CREAM (both from ProCyte) and/or chilled 100% Aloe Vera Gel after every treatment. This can greatly reduce the risk of blisters and will heal the skin more quickly.
- I also recommend having SILVER SULFADIAZINE CREAM USP 1% on hand. Only use this if you see immediate burns
- You must also apply a good, full spectrum sun protection on areas that will be even moderately exposed to the sun. I recommend TI-SILC SHEER SPF45 (from ProCyte).
- On a final note, you can also offer small ice packs to the patient to take home if they are feeling very warm. I order mine with my company logo on it.

You can find contact information for ProCyte, Creative Technologies and Palomar in the Resource and References Chapter 21

Testimonials

To help you better understand what treatments feel like and what they can do for you, I have included the following excerpts from Thank You letters and testimonials from my patients:

Dear Laura,

Divine Laser showed me that it is possible to bring out your inner beauty, not only because of their magnificent treatments, but also because of the good and warm treatment of the people who apply their valuable experience to you.

—B.C.

* * * * * * * * * * * *

Hi Laura,

Divine Laser is a dream. I have experienced an amazing difference after only two treatments. My skin around my bikini line became softer and smoother with each treatment. I no longer have that next-day, course razor stubble that is inevitable with shaving. I look forward to every treatment because the results are so remarkable. I have tried laser treatments from other places and found their processes to be painful and unnoticeable. I have recommended Divine Laser to all of my friends. I have friends that are willing to fly to Phoenix to experience the results that I have. The staff is also so wonderful—professional, skilled and friendly.

—Paula

* * * * * * * * * * * *

Dear Laura,

My experience was relaxing and rejuvenating. Thanks to the entire staff for making my visit so comfortable. I especially appreciate the privacy of the environment—being a female who wears makeup almost all the time, having your face bare can be uncomfortable—the setting at Divine Laser is cozy and private. Thanks again for helping me— it has changed my life! I hope this sums up how I feel about my experience. I will see you all soon for my next visit.

Have a super day!
—Shelley B.

(P.S. Remember, if you smile, all your wrinkles
will be in the right places—ha,ha,ha!)

* * * * * * * * * * * *

Dear Laura and the Divine Staff,

THANK YOU, THANK YOU, THANK YOU!!!!!!! I am writing to tell you how DIVINELY HAPPY you have made me. Your products and services are changing my life!

—J.M.C.

* * * * * * * * * * * *

Dear Laura and The Divinely Divine Staff at Divine,
In October I stopped by Divine Laser with a friend. My intention was to ask about BOTOX® Cosmetic. Before I knew it, I was asking Divine Laser's owner, Laura Regan, and members of her fully trained staff of professionals about skin care, products, makeup and hair removal! For the first time in a long time, I felt that someone (besides me) REALLY CARED about helping me. That meant the world to me! Instead of making me purchase products right away, Laura GAVE me samples to try with specific instructions. She actually took time out (free of charge) to educate me. I eventually purchased the products that she recommended and also received a few of the treatments, and I AM A NEW PERSON! Thank you for helping me feel good about myself again. I LOVE Divine Laser Hair Removal and Skin Care.

—Jane

* * * * * * * * * * * *

To the "Laser Queen"—
You are amazing. Visiting Divine Laser was the best experience I have had in a long time. You are dedicated to your profession and you are so concerned, that it was very surprising. I have suffered (literally) from facial hair my entire life. You understand how I feel, and that made all the difference in the world. I used to hold my head down, and now I hold it up proudly…because of you! You were truly a DIVINE INTERVENTION for me.

Thank you— A—

* * * * * * * * * * * *

To Laura at Divine Laser:
Thank you—thank you—thank you—thank you—thank you! It took many years, but I finally talked my husband into removing his "back shirt." He was so hesitant, but he said you

made him so comfortable and you were so nice and understanding. He has had GREAT results and he is a new man now! I send you a million THANK YOUs!!!!!!

—**Tammy T.**

* * * * * * * * * * * *

Hi Laura!

I can't believe the difference you have made in my husband's appearance. He suffered terribly from severe razor rash and ingrown hairs on his beard and neck. Even after just the first treatment, he no longer complains about the problem. He is so happy and is telling all his friends. He had a wonderful experience and he is insisting that I sign up for a package as well, so I will see you next week. You are the "Hair Removal Queen"!!!

* * * * * * * * * * * *

To Divine Laser,

{The treatments] are so worth the minor discomfort. I am upset that I didn't start treatments earlier. I love the results. It has given me a greater sense of sexual confidence.

* * * * * * * * * * * *

Dear Laura,

I can't believe I waited so many years to have this done! I am so happy that at 40 I am finally hairless and unburdened with shaving every day. You warned me in the beginning that this was addictive, and you were right! Our relationship lasted almost two years because I kept adding areas. At this point, I don't shave my underarms, bikini area or legs AT ALL anymore. I calculated my time savings and it is roughly 7,300 hours per year (I would spend at least 15 to 25 minutes EVERY DAY shaving these areas, as well as tediously tweezing my chin and neck). I don't think you realize what this has done for my life. The quality of my life has so dra-

matically improved that my husband and even my children notice "something different" about me. I can hardly explain it because the feeling is so intense. Can you believe I am going to actually miss my treatments?! At first, I was so shy and timid and even scared of what it would feel like. By the second treatment, I was shocked at just how EASY the sensation was compared to waxing. That cold roller was a lifesaver. I never thought I would be able to sit through the full leg treatment, but using the cooling technique was a true blessing. The worst I ever felt was like I had a sunburn, but the results are so worth it. Again, my one and only regret is that I did not do this YEARS ago. I definitely would have been a different person back then. I am so thankful to you and your hard work. You were always so understanding—right from the very first treatment. I remember how gentle you were and how you calmed me down. When you told me that you had the same problem (facial and excessive body hair), I immediately felt assured that I was in the right hands. I could not believe that I was not alone! Saying "thank you" is not even close to being enough (my husband is very pleased with your one-of-a-kind bikini sculpting as well...run the other way if you see him because he said he would hug and kiss you if he ran into you!). I am so excited about your book, and I hope this letter can give you some important feedback for it. If I had a book that detailed everything that you told me will be in it, I probably would have been diagnosed with my PCOS (same as you again!) so long ago. I would have saved years of torment, pain, depression and confusion. I hope your book will help women better understand and LISTEN to their bodies.

I wish you all the best! Thank you for a new, smoother, happier me!

—Anonymous

CHAPTER 15

(Courtesy of SkinMedica Inc.)
SPECIAL ISSUES IN TREATING
PATIENTS OF COLOR

"Where The Determination Is, The Way Can Be Found."
—George S. Clason, *The Richest Man In Babylon*

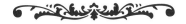

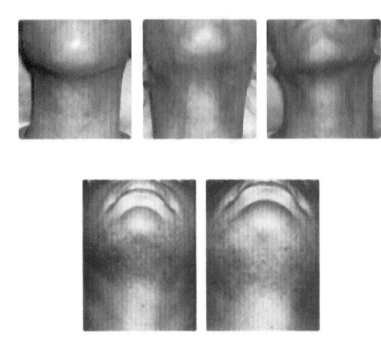

Excessive facial hair in patients of color (defined here as Fitzpatrick skin types IV-VI) is frequently complicated by the co-existence of pseudofolliculitus (PFB), post-inflammatory hyper-pigmentation, (PIH) (excess, darker pigment)and keloids which may result from attempts to remove unwanted hair. Significantly more Melanin absorption occurs in individuals of color, which increases the risk of epidermal damage. Extra care must be taken when treating patients of color with lasers to prevent pigmentary changes, irritation and blistering.

In my experience, the combination of IPL treatments and use of Vaniqa® cream is the best option for patients with dark skin. So keep in mind that if you have dark (or consistently tan skin) which is Fitzpatrick IV-VI, "regular" lasers are not for you. You will need to search for a facility that offers and advertises treatments for dark skin (most likely they will use IPL).

KEYPOINT: It is a good idea to get "test spots" before you begin (and pay for) a treatment of any kind. You should receive a few "hits" at a few different levels (the technician will decide on the levels) in or around the actual area that you want to treat. You should wait at least 72 hours to see exactly what happens to the skin. If there are no problems, you will feel more confident about beginning treatment.

CHAPTER 16

TROUBLESHOOTING: *Why Am I Not Getting Results?*

"If at first you don't succeed, you're
running about average."
—M.H. Alderson

Some patients see results after just one treatment, while others don't start to see any results until their fourth or fifth treatment. It is important to understand that we all are unique and we are all different. This fact plays a huge role in determining how quickly we achieve results. There are no guarantees or set "rules" to follow when it comes to a specific result timeline. You have to go into each treatment with an open mind. After reading this book, you now know that laser/IPL procedures are used to permanently reduce hair (not completely remove it forever). You have also learned about many things that can complicate the process and even delay progress. Over the years I had some patients tell me, "This is going to be my fourth treatment and hair is still growing. This isn't working." In so many of these cases, I did an analysis of their treatment intervals and clearly reviewed their adherence to the pre- and post-care instructions. We discussed it, revised a few things, or simply just waited it out and did a few more treatments.

In *most* of these cases, patients did receive some form of permanent hair reduction and were somewhat satisfied.

> **KEYPOINT: If you are dissatisfied with your results, talk to your technician or provider. Be completely honest about what you are doing in-between treatments. Maybe you just need to get treatments eight weeks apart instead of six; maybe you interrupted progress by tweezing or waxing; or maybe you have a disorder that needs medical attention. You have to take everything into consideration. DON'T GIVE UP! You must keep educating yourself, be committed to the process, and be patient.**

Here are some fabricated scenarios and some possible options. In most cases, my options or solutions include my favorite phrases: "set realistic expectations"; "be committed"; "be consistent"; "be patient"; "persevere!"

A) You are not getting results **WHAT IS GOING ON?**

You have not followed pre-or post-care instructions properly and you waxed and plucked the treatment area in-between treatments.

B) You received your second treatment on your bikini line seven days ago. You see what looks like full growth. **WHAT IS GOING ON?** It is called "push out." The hairs under the skin at the time of treatment are now pushing themselves out of their follicles. It is not new growth.

C) You signed up for five sessions of IPL treatments on your upper lip. Your provider recommended treatments three weeks apart. You have followed all pre- and post-care instructions and faithfully received treatments exactly three weeks apart as directed. It is now two weeks after your fourth treatment and you look in the mirror and see hair growth on your lip as if you had never received a treatment. **WHAT IS GOING ON?** The treatment intervals recommended by providers are "guesstimates." Your particular growth cycle might be four weeks instead of three weeks (SEE PAGE 157 FOR MORE DETAILS).

D) You have had two treatments on your entire face so far. You were told to shave before each treatment and in-between if necessary. You notice that the hairs have gotten thinner and lighter. **WHAT SHOULD YOU DO?** Actually, it is good that the hairs are getting thinner and lighter because it means that the treatments are working. Unfortunately, it also means that the progress of results can slow down a bit because lighter, finer hairs are harder to kill (this is kind of a catch-22 situation).

> **KEYPOINT: You have to stick with it—stay committed and persevere! You can also add Vaniqa® to your treatment plan to help slow down the regrowth. Different**

196

> **areas tend to receive different results. Often, areas on the face are more difficult to treat due to many factors (like hormones, curved follicles, lighter hairs) as opposed to the bikini area which often has dark, thick hair and responds to treatment faster.**

E) You have been diagnosed with PCOS. You decided to go on birth control pills and start IPL or laser treatments. After three months (and three laser treatments), you still seem to have the same amount of facial hair. **WHAT IS GOING ON?** When you have a disorder that causes hair growth, it is much more difficult to kill the hairs, and you must go into treatment understanding that. You are fighting a tougher battle. Also, new hair might start to grow as you kill off other hair, so it appears as though you are not getting results. The birth control pills can take many months to start to work, so patience is required. I would also recommend adding Vaniqa® to your treatment plan (COMBINATION THERAPY). Vaniqa® can slow down the regrowth of hairs in-between laser treatments. Vaniqa® can also take a few months to start working, so even more patience is required.

F) You completed a total of nine laser treatments on your chin and neck. The last treatment was two years ago. The results were great and you have enjoyed smoothness. Only some fine, light hairs remained. Then, you suddenly notice about five or six dark hairs pop out on your chin. **WHAT SHOULD YOU DO?** You have learned in this book that the number of hair follicles we have is predetermined at birth. We have dormant follicles and active follicles. During your entire treatment process, only the active follicles were destroyed. More than likely, those six hairs that recently popped out are completely new hairs (from the follicles that were dormant during your laser treatments). This can continue to happen in the future as well. DO NOT start to pluck or wax. Simply get what I call a "touch-up" laser or IPL treatment. I also recommend starting to use Vaniqa® at this point (see Chapter 17) to slow down the growth (this worked great for me). Also, you can use Meladine™ (see Chapter 18) to dye the lighter hairs to kill them off, so you are not bothered by the light hairs and achieve an even smoother result (this also worked great for me!).

G) After three IPL treatments, it actually looks like you have the same if not MORE hair than you started with! **WHAT IS GOING ON?** Although this theory is highly unlikely, check with your provider about the setting used on you for all of your treatments. Treatments performed on an excessively low setting can actually stimulate hair growth. The more reasonable explanation is that you are seeing a "massive push out." I have seen this many, many times. As long as the patient's skin is capable of tolerating a high setting (without risk of burns), I put them on the highest setting they can take for the next few treatments, and results start to kick in. *I have them watch their growth cycle VERY closely for the next few treatments as well. In summary, you want to be sure you are treating as many hairs in the anagen cycle on the highest level as possible.

KEYPOINT: Hirsutism is a very complicated condition. Unfortunately, trying to achieve permanent results can be even more complicated! Results do not happen overnight. Remember: Have realistic expectations; educate yourself; be consistent; be patient; be committed; follow pre- and post-care instructions and persevere! This book is a valuable tool and what you learn throughout these pages is valuable. Use the information to your benefit. Good luck and don't give up!

CHAPTER 17

VANIQA®: THE VANISHING ACT
(*courtesy of SkinMedica, Inc.*)

"Vaniqa® really works, especially when used
in conjunction with IPL treatments."
—Anonymous (Patient)

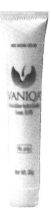

Eighty-one percent of women with UFH self-treat their condition. Many product and treatments options are available. Vaniqa® is the only prescription product clinically proven to slow the growth of UFH. However, Vaniqa® does not stop the growth of UFH. Therefore, it must be used in conjunction with a hair removal method in order to achieve best results (See "Combination Therapy" Chapter 19). When Vaniqa® is used in addition to an effective method of hair removal (or reduction), women report a significant reduction in the time spent removing, treating and concealing UFH.

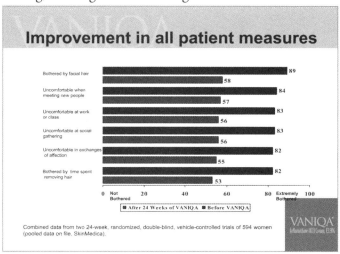

In my personal opinion, Vaniqa® is an exceptional product. I personally started using Vaniqa® many years ago. Throughout the years, I have incorporated Vaniqa® into many case studies, and the results and findings have been nothing short of amazing. I was deeply frustrated when it came to treating gray, white and blond hair—especially when I was treating women and transgender patients who suffered from hirsutism on the face and were desperate for help. After dozens of case studies with these patients, I found that incorporating Vaniqa® into my IPL treatment plan made the difference I was looking for. The IPL treatments did their job and treated the dark hairs, and Vaniqa® picked up the "slack" and slowed down the growth of the light hairs as well as the dark hairs (*see Chapter 19 to learn more about "Combination Therapies"*).

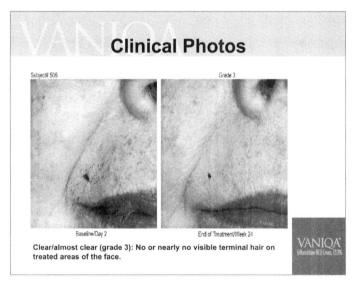

What is Vaniqa®?

Vaniqa®, a cream containing 13.9 percent (139 milligrams/gram) of eflornithine (Eh-FLOR-ni-theen) hydrochloride (HCI), is

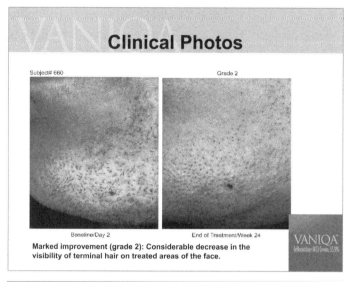

Marked improvement (grade 2): Considerable decrease in the visibility of terminal hair on treated areas of the face.

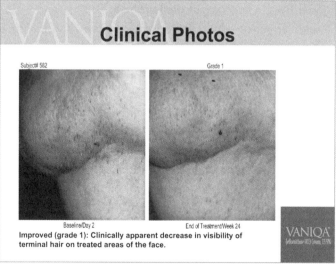

Improved (grade 1): Clinically apparent decrease in visibility of terminal hair on treated areas of the face.

indicated for the reduction of unwanted facial hair (UFH) in women. Vaniqa® is indicated for use only on the face, as studies have not been done on other areas of the body. Vaniqa® is a prescription drug product, supplied in a 30-gram tube.

Vaniqa® (eflornithine hydrochloride) Cream, 13.9 percent has demonstrated significant improvement in reduction of facial hair in several well-controlled clinical trials.

History of Vaniqa®

Eflornithine HCI was previously known as alphadifluoromethylornithine, or DFMO. An oral form of eflornithine was initially developed in the late 1970s at Merrell Dow Research Institute as an anticancer therapy. However, the compound was not effective as a single therapeutic agent. In the early 1980s, an injectable form of eflornithine was licensed to the World Health Organization for the treatment of African Sleeping Sickness (ASS), and in 1990, eflornithine was approved by the FDA as an orphan drug.

A side effect of eflornithine treatment was significant hair loss. A formulation patent was filed by Gillette in 1997 on topical eflornithine cream for hair growth inhibition. In a cooperative development/marketing effort, Bristol-Myers Squibb filed a New Drug Application (NDA) for eflornithine HCI (cream) in 1999, which gained FDA approval in July 2000. SkinMedica acquired the marketing rights to Vaniqa® in 2004, complementing their prescription skin care product line. International marketing rights are held by Shire Pharmaceuticals.

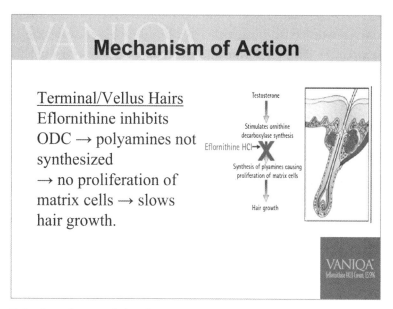

Mechanism of Action

The active ingredient of Vaniqa®, eflornithine HCl, is an irreversible inhibitor of the enzyme, ornithine decarboxylase (ODC). ODC is one of a family of enzymes which facilitate the synthesis of compounds called polyamines which, in the skin, stimulate follicular development and subsequent terminal hair formation. Androgens, such as testosterone, increase ODC activity, not only in skin, but also in other organs such as the testis and the prostate, which undergo masculine differentiation at adolescence. ODC is known to be present in the follicular bulb and hair shaft.

During anagen (growth phase), ODC is responsible for stimulating polyamines to "cue" the germinal matrix cells to produce terminal hair shaft proteins. When eflornithine is present, this process is interrupted (ODC inhibition) and hair growth is slowed.

ODC is continually manufactured in the hair follicle during the growth phase (anagen), so inhibition by eflornithine is temporary. Thus, eflornithine treatment does not arrest hair growth, but merely slows it. Eflornithine is only effective during anagen, when ODC is active. Hair which is not in anagen at the time of treatment will not be affected. Therefore, eflornithine (Vaniqa®) must be continuously applied in order to maintain growth inhibition of anagen hairs and assure an effect on follicles transitioning into the growth phase. Studies have shown that if Vaniqa® is discontinued, hair will return to pretreatment condition in about eight weeks.

Vaniqa® Dosage and Administration

- Vaniqa® is NOT a hair remover. Vaniqa® is not meant to replace but rather should be used in conjunction with a woman's current method of hair removal.

- Even though eflornithine HCI is believed to be an irreversible inhibitor of ODC, the enzyme is continually regenerating. Therefore, it is necessary for women to apply Vaniqa® twice daily in order to continue to see results.

- Apply a thin layer of Vaniqa® to affected areas of the face and also to adjacent involved areas. Rub in thoroughly. Do not wash treated area for at least four hours. Use twice daily at least eight hours apart or as directed by a physician.

- Vaniqa® should be applied at least five minutes after hair removal.

- Vaniqa® should be used every day, but it is not necessary for consumers to remove hair every time they apply Vaniqa®.

> - If irritation occurs, frequency of treatment should be reduced. If irritation persists, Vaniqa® should be discontinued.

Side Effects (Adverse Events)

When side effects occurred, they were mild and generally resolved without treatment. The most common side effects associated with Vaniqa® included minor skin irritations such as temporary redness, hair bumps or razor bumps (pseudofolliculitis barbae), stinging, burning, tingling, acne or rash.

A higher incidence of acne in both treatment groups may have been a result of the shaving required by the protocol. Many of these patients were shaving for the first time. In normal use, consumers using a hair removal method should continue to do so; they are not required to shave.

Only two percent of subjects in Vaniqa® studies discontinued treatment due to an adverse event related to Vaniqa®.

It is not known if Vaniqa® has any interactions with other topically applied drug products. Cosmetics or sunscreens may be applied over treated areas after Vaniqa® has dried.

If skin irritation or intolerance develops with Vaniqa® use, the patient should be directed to reduce application frequency to once daily. If irritation continues, the patient should discontinue use of the product.

How Do I Get Vaniqa®?

Vaniqa® is a prescription cream. Consult with your doctor or laser/IPL professional.

Vaniqa® Testimonials

❖ Jane, Female, Age 57

"I tried Vaniqa® about five years ago, but I got lazy and I didn't continue applying the cream every day. My condition worsened, and before I knew it, I had a beard (at least it felt like it). Three years ago, I had a series of five laser treatments. My condition improved, but I still had growth. I did some research and found a laser specialist that combined these two therapies together. I signed up for another series of five treatments. Although the results did not take place overnight, by the end of my five treatments, I was very, very satisfied with the outcome. I owe it all to using laser and IPL in conjunction with one another."

❖ Anonymous, Female, Age 26

"I have PCOS. After a few laser treatments, all I noticed was a reduction in the amount of hair on my face and chest. My laser technician recommended that I also start using Vaniqa®. After a few months, I noticed a big difference. I would still have to shave after my treatments, but then I would be smooth for weeks. I have completed a total of nine IPL treatments, and I don't even have to shave at all anymore. My life is changed. I still use Vaniqa®, however. I love the way it makes my face feel. The cream is very smooth and moisturizing. I only have to apply it a few times a week now, so it is easy to keep up with. My skin looks great, and I am using the Vaniqa® to maintain the finer, lighter hair that I have left on my face. I am very happy."

❖ Lynne T., Female, Age 33

"I love Vaniqa®. My face really does feel nice and soft when I use it. I had a lot of blond hair on my face and it really bothered me. Since I was not a candidate for laser, I decided to use Vaniqa®. It has really slowed down the growth, and my husband even noticed the difference!"

❖ Anonymous, Male Transsexual, Age 38

"The final step in a very long ordeal for me was getting rid of my facial hair. Hormone therapy only did so much. I had so many laser treatments over the years, but I just never got the results I was looking for. My doctor referred me to a laser specialist and she recommended combination therapy. All I can say is WOW. It is truly a miracle, and I feel so complete now. I almost gave up because it did take a few months to start working. Then one day, I had my hand on my face and all I felt was smooth skin. I realized that I had not shaved in, like, five days. That was a first for me. It has gotten better and better ever since. I am close to a point where I hardly shave at all. Words cannot explain my joy. Combination therapy is a lifesaver!"

❖ T.T., Male, Age 64

"I have tried everything to get rid of the hair on my ears. I spent so much money over the years and nothing worked, even laser treatments. I was so disappointed. I expressed this to my doctor on just a regular visit for a check up. He prescribed Vaniqa® for me. I used it religiously, and in about two months, I noticed that not only were my ears less hairy, but my skin felt smooth. It is hard to explain, but the smoothness was more than just the decrease in hair. It has been a year since I started it. Now I only put the cream on one to two times a week. It is so easy and I actually like using it. I told everyone I know about it. Now, all the guys at the golf club are avid Vaniqa® users!"

CHAPTER 18

CHALLENGING THE TOUGHEST ENEMY: BLOND, GRAY AND WHITE HAIR

"Believe you are defeated. Believe it long enough, and it is likely to become a fact."
—Norman Vincent Peale

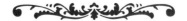

Throughout my years of service in the permanent hair reduc
tion industry, I have tried almost every product known to man
to combat light hair (blond, gray, white and true red). Red hair
has been my toughest struggle. Lasers and IPL cannot pick up
(or kill) true red hair. The color red is not captured within the
wavelength spectrum.

In my business of IPL permanent hair reduction, it is very
difficult to offer a service that does not include light or red
hair. Many patients spend a lot of time and money on IPL
treatments, only to be left with some light hairs. Or, on the flip
side, there are many patients who have either true red hair or all
gray, white or blond hair and are ruled out completely. It is so
disappointing. Luckily, after months of research, I realized that
there are only a few viable options (this is strictly my opinion).

Option #1—Meladine™

Meladine™ is a natural melanin enhancer (*Courtesy of
Creative Technologies, Inc., Chesapeake, VA 23320).

As we have learned, lasers and IPL treatments use the naturally occurring melanin in the hair follicle as a target to
selectively disable the follicle while leaving surrounding skin
structures intact. However, lighter hair either has too little
melanin or the wrong type of melanin to provide an effective
target for the laser, so people with white, gray and blond hair
have not been suitable candidates for laser hair removal.
Meladine™ offers a viable option for these patients.

When sprayed on the desired area, Meladine™'s™ patent-
ed liposome delivery system selectively deposits natural melanin
directly into the hair follicle without staining surrounding skin.
The proprietary liposome molecules are small enough to effectively penetrate the infundibulum (hair follicle), but are not
taken up by the bloodstream. The result is temporary melanin-rich

follicles [Figure 1], which allow patients with lighter hair colors to benefit from laser hair removal.

> **KEYPOINT: I have used Meladine™ for the remaining fine, light hairs on my face. The process is time-consuming and tedious. So you must be committed and follow the instructions diligently. You will only achieve results if you are consistent.**

Suggested Use for Fine, Soft, Vellus Hair

1. Begin your daily Meladine™ routine 14 days prior to each laser treatment.

2. It is important that the hair be shaved or clipped daily. Do NOT wax, tweeze or use depilatories on the area between treatments.

3. Always apply Meladine™ to clean skin. Do not use cosmetic preparations prior to application of Meladine™.

4. In the morning, spray the area to be treated with Meladine™ and allow to dry. Repeat this spraying and drying process four to six times. It is imperative that Meladine™ be allowed to dry between each spray. Hold sprayer three to five inches away from area to be treated.

5. Research has indicated that gently patting the Meladine™ into the skin before drying can help with absorption.

6. Repeat step 4 in the evening.

Note: For maximum results, product must be used as directed daily for a minimum of 14 days prior to treatment. Results may vary depending on proper use, patient compliance and other variable factors.

Store in a cool, dry place. Refrigeration is recommended for storage of Meladine™ between laser treatments.

Suggested use for coarse, gray or white hair:

1) Follow the same as above except you must use it for a longer period of time to penetrate the thicker hairs. Begin your **daily** Meladine™ routine **four to six weeks prior** to each laser treatment.

*Steps 2—6 same as above

> **KEYPOINT: After each spraying session, you will then receive laser or IPL treatments. It is common to use the product for months, with up to 9 or 10 laser or IPL treatments before seeing results.**

How long does one bottle last?

One bottle contains approximately 720 sprays, which may be enough to cover several regimens (regimen = series of applications prior to one laser treatment) for a lip, but may only cover one regimen for a full face. The duration of one bottle will be determined by several factors:

1) Size of the area to be treated: Obviously smaller areas will require less product. A lip may require one spray to sufficiently cover the area per application, while a back may require six to eight sprays per application.

2) Type of hair to be treated: Patients treating fine, vellus hair (two weeks of use prior to laser treatment) will use less product than patients treating coarse hair (six weeks of use prior to laser treatment) because the application regimen is shorter.

3) Patient preference: Some patients may apply Meladine™ more liberally per application.

I treat quite a few patients with Meladine™. Results will be achieved only with a strong and consistent commitment to the entire processes involved. It takes perseverance and patience. It does not happen overnight (as with most things in life). There are no guarantees, and there are so many variables involved that results can take a long time. The end result in most cases I have dealt with have been worth it. So, if you are serious about hair removal and you are truly determined to finally get rid of excessive or unwanted "light" hairs, this can be a good option for you. I must reiterate the following words: **CONSISTENCE, COMMITMENT, PERSERVERANCE** and **PATIENCE!**

*If this tedious process is not for you—don't worry—you still have some more options!

OPTION #2—ELECTROLYSIS (See Chapter 7 for more details.)

OPTION #3—VANIQA® (See Chapter 17.)

OPTION #4—"COMBINATION THERAPY"—Electrolysis treatments "combined" with Vaniqa® and/or Meladine™ and laser/IPL. (See Chapter 19 for details.)

CHAPTER 19

THE ULTIMATE BATTLE PLAN:
COMBINATION THERAPY

"You may have to fight a battle more than once to win it."
—Margaret Thatcher

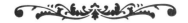

Combination therapy is when you combine two or more cosmetic treatments *or* when you combine cosmetic and systemic therapies. You have to treat the inside and the outside for a total recovery.

If you are diagnosed with a disorder that is causing hirsutism, you will most likely receive medical therapy to regulate your hormone levels. Once a treatment has proven to be effective, it is continued indefinitely. Because it is usually not possible to cure the hormonal problem causing the excess hair growth, hirsutism will return if medical treatment is stopped. Unfortunately, medical therapies do not remove the hair you already have. Therefore, you must *combine* your medical therapy with a form of permanent hair reduction such as laser or IPL treatments. Doing just one or the other will not give you the "smoothness" you are looking for. A person with a specific disorder (like PCOS) can receive numerous IPL or laser treatments but they wont get REAL, LASTING results until they take care of the disorder and decrease the CAUSE of the hair growth!

I have also learned over the past several years that in many cases, "smooth" results are significantly improved and accelerated if we *combine* hair removal methods as well. There are so many options available. You have learned about treatment options in Chapter 7, so you can see just how many options you have. Your doctor can help you decide on a game plan.

After years of research and completing case studies on patients with specific disorders (like PCOS), my combination of choice is:

1) Follow your doctor's prescription orders for systemic therapy (medication) OR natural hormone therapy.

2) Begin Intense Pulsed Light (IPL) treatments.

3) *Incorporate Meladine™ if you have a majority of blond, gray, red or white hair.

4) Enhance the results by using Vaniqa® throughout your IPL treatment course.

5) Use electrolysis as a "touch-up" method to help kill off stray "light" hairs.

The most common protocol my patients follow is the IPL/Vaniqa® therapy. The IPL treatments permanently reduce the amount of hair you have, and Vaniqa® slows down the regrowth so you have smoother skin (for longer periods of time) between IPL treatments.

> **KEYPOINT: If you incorporate Vaniqa® into your laser or IPL treatment plan, you MUST take into consideration that Vaniqa® will SLOW DOWN the regrowth. Therefore, you must adjust your treatment intervals. The time frame for the entire treatment course can increase significantly. (If you are treating a chin and would normally treat the patient every 3 weeks, you would probably increase that to 4 or even as much as 8 weeks when using Vaniqa®. Therefore, the entire course for 8 IPL treatments would normally take approximately 28-30 weeks)will take 58 or more weeks with the addition of Vaniqa®**

Laser/IPL and Vaniqa®

According to research from Vaniqa® and SkinMedica, Inc., women show statistically greater preference for Vaniqa® in combination with their standard hair removal method compared to standard hair removal alone. Vaniqa® clinical-trials data demonstrated significant reduction in how bothered women felt by their facial hair and the time they spent treating it.

Studies of Vaniqa® in Combination with Laser Hair Removal

Two Phase IV clinical trials have studied the effects of Vaniqa ® as adjunct therapy to laser/IPL hair removal. One study was conducted in Canada by investigators at the University of British Columbia, Division of Dermatology, and the other was conducted in the U.S. through the University of California, San Diego, Division of Dermatology. Both studies used randomized, double-blind, vehicle-controlled study designs. In both studies, both sides of the face were subjected to laser/IPL hair removal treatment, after which one side of the face received vehicle cream and the other side was treated with Vaniqa®. The treated (Vaniqa®) and control (laser plus cream vehicle) were compared.

Laser or IPL and Vaniqa® Clinical-Trials Summary

As previously discussed, using Vaniqa® as adjunct to laser/IPL treatment has been definitively demonstrated in controlled clinical trials to enhance the rate and degree of hair removal. Both studies were right/left bilateral face studies, wherein laser/IPL was applied to both sides of the face and Vaniqa® was applied to one side only.

One study found that after 6 months of once-a-month laser/IPL treatment and twice daily use of Vaniqa®, 27 out of 28 patients (96.4 percent) had complete or almost complete removal of UFH compared to 19 out of 28 patients (67.9 percent) treated with laser/IPL alone. Hair counts were decreased 89 percent for laser plus Vaniqa® compared to an 80 percent decrease for laser plus vehicle $(f<0.01)$.

The other study (22) demonstrated a significant reduction in hair growth for Vaniqa® plus laser at post-treatment weeks 6 through 10. Laser/IPL treatment was performed only twice at weeks 2 and 10. Side effects were minimal and of similar nature and frequency for laser/IPL and laser/IPL plus Vaniqa® patients.

In conclusion, the efficacy and safety of hair removal is constantly improving with advancements in laser and pulsed light technologies. Widespread use of these systems is availing them to a broader segment of the population, thereby opening up an extraordinary opportunity for the SkinMedica sales force to educate physicians on the synergistic combination of laser/IPL and Vaniqa® and reinforce the significant benefits of Vaniqa® use with all methods of hair removal.

> **KEYPOINT: It is time to alleviate psychosocial fears and inhibitions associated with UFH, by raising public awareness of the availability of safe and efficacious management methods. The addition of Vaniqa® to all hair removal treatments takes a significant step toward achieving a scientifically sound, long-term solution to the burden of UFH.**

CHAPTER 20

GLOSSARY OF TERMS

- **Absorption**—The taking in or incorporation of something, such as a gas, a liquid, light or heat.
- **Acanthosis Nigricans**—An eruption of velvety wartlike growths accompanied by hyperpigmentation in the skin of the armpits, neck, anogenital area and groin, occurring in a benign form in children but associated with internal malignancy or reticulosis in adults.
- **Accutane**—A trademark used for the drug isotretinoin.
- **Isotretinoin** is a generic medication used for the treatment of severe _acne_ and is most commonly known under the brands **Accutane** and **Roaccutane**. It is a _retinoid,_ meaning it is derived from vitamin A and is found naturally in the body, produced by the liver in small quantities.
- **Acne**—An inflammatory disease of the sebaceous glands and hair follicles of the skin that is marked by the eruption of pimples or pustules, especially on the face.
- **Actinic Bronzing**—Diffuse browning of the skin.
- **Adrenal Gland**—Either of two small, dissimilarly shaped endocrine glands, one located above each kidney, consisting of the cortex, which secretes several steroid hormones, and the medulla, which secretes epinephrine. Also called **suprarenal gland**.
- **Alpha-Hydroxy**—Alpha-Hydroxy acids (AHAs) are naturally occurring carbolic acids. Glycolic acid, the most commonly recognized and advertised AHA, is derived from sugar cane.
- **Anagen**—The growth stage of hair development.
- **Analogies**—Similarity in some respects between things that are otherwise dissimilar; a comparison based on such similarity.
- **Analysis**—The separation of an intellectual or material whole into its constituent parts for individual study; the study of such constituent parts and their interrelationships in making up a whole.
- **Androgen**—Hormones, such as testosterone and dihydrotestosterone, responsible for the development of male characteristics. In women, androgen is produced in small amounts in the ovaries and adrenal glands. These hormones are necessary for normal sex drives.
- **Androgenic**—A steroid hormone, such as testosterone or androsterone, that controls the development and maintenance of masculine characteristics. Also called **androgenic hormone**.
- **Androstenedione**—An unsaturated androgenic steroid existing in three isomeric forms that is secreted by the testis, ovaries and adrenal cortex and has a weaker biological potency than testosterone.
- **Annoyed**—To cause slight irritation to (another) by troublesome, often-repeated acts; to harass or disturb by repeated attacks.
- **Antisocial**—Shunning the society of others; not sociable; hostile to or

disruptive of the established social order; marked by or engaging in behavior that violates accepted mores: *gangs engaging in vandalism and other antisocial behavior;* antagonistic toward or disrespectful of others; rude.

- **Antivirals**—Destroying or inhibiting the growth and reproduction of viruses.
- **Anxiety**—A state of uneasiness and apprehension, as about future uncertainties.
- **Anxious** (in social situations)—Uneasy and apprehensive about an uncertain event or matter; worried.
- **Apocrine Glands**—Responsible for your body odor.
- **Aquaphor**—Aquaphor Healing Ointment protects dry, cracked or irritated skin to help enhance the natural healing process and restore smooth, healthy skin.
- **Arrector Pili**—A muscle attached to a hair follicle. In response to cold temperatures or fear, the muscle contracts, pulling the hair upright and dimpling the skin surface (goose bumps).
- **Axillary Hair**—Coarse strands of hair; found mainly around the nipples and under the arms (armpits).
- **Beastly**—Of or resembling a beast; bestial.
- **Biochemical**—Of or relating to biochemistry; involving chemical processes in living organisms.
- **Bio-Identical Hormones**—*Bio-Identical Natural Hormones (BNHs) are hormones that are molecularly (biochemically) identical to your true major ovarian steroid hormones—progesterone, estradiol and testosterone. They are derived from a Natural source—soybean or yam, and are Bioidentical to your ovarian Hormones—thus, the name Bioidentical Natural Hormones (BNHs).*
- **Blistering**—A local swelling of the skin that contains watery fluid and is caused by burning or irritation.
- **Catagen**—The transition phase in the hair growth cycle, in which growth (anagen) stops and resting (telogen) begins.
- **Cause**—The one, such as a person, event or condition, that is responsible for an action or result.
- **Chromophore**—A chemical group capable of selective light absorption resulting in the coloration of certain organic compounds.
- **Chronic**—Lasting for a long period of time or marked by frequent recurrence, as certain diseases.
- **Clinical**—Involving or based on direct observation of the patient.
- **Commitment**—A pledge to do.
- **Complex Cu3**—ProCyte's Complex Cu3 products are enhanced with

GHK Copper Peptide Complex to feed the skin with copper micro-nutrition. Complex Cu3 provides patients with a total skin care system to ensure an optimal post-procedure healing environment.

- **Compound**—To combine so as to form a whole; mix.
- **Condition**—A mode or state of being.
- **Congenial**—Having the same tastes, habits or temperament; sympathetic.
- **Conjunction**—The act of joining; the state of being joined.
- **Contraindications**—A factor that precludes the administration of a drug or the carrying out of a medical procedure.
- **Cortex**—The region of tissue in a root or stem lying between the epidermis and the vascular tissue.
- **Corticosteroids**—Medication that can prevent the adrenal gland from producing androgens.
- **Cortisol**—An adrenal-cortex hormone (trade names Hydrocortone or Cortef) that is active in carbohydrate and protein metabolism.
- **Cross-Dresser**—One who dresses in clothing characteristic of the opposite sex.
- **Cuticle**—The outermost layer of the skin of vertebrates; epidermis.
- **Cyclic**—Of, relating to, or characterized by cycles.
- **Cyclosporine**—An immunosuppressive drug obtained from certain soil fungi, used mainly to prevent the rejection of transplanted organs.
- **Dehydroepiandrosterone**—An androgenic ketosteroid secreted by the adrenal cortex that is an intermediate in the biosynthesis of testosterone.
- **Depression**—A psychiatric disorder characterized by an inability to concentrate, insomnia, loss of appetite, anhedonia, feelings of extreme sadness, guilt, helplessness and hopelessness, and thoughts of death. Also called **clinical depression.**
- **Dermal**—Of or relating to the skin or dermis.
- **Dermal Papilla**—Any of the superficial projections of the corium or dermis that interlock with recesses in the overlying epidermis, contain vascular loops and specialized nerve endings, and are arranged in ridge-like lines most prominent in the hand and foot. Also called *papilla of corium.*
- **Dermatologist**—A medical professional who specializes in the physiology and pathology of the skin.
- **Dermatology**—The branch of medicine that is concerned with the physiology and pathology of the skin.
- **Dermis**—The second layer of skin where most skin appendages are located; the dermis is primarily comprised of connective tissue— collagen and elastin.

- **Desperate**—Having lost all hope; despairing.
- **Dihydrotestosterone**—Active form of testosterone in the skin.
- **Disadvantaged**—An unfavorable condition or circumstance.
- **Dormant**—Lying asleep or as if asleep; inactive.
- **Double-Blind**—With respect to clinical trials, a test in which neither the patient nor the study personnel know which treatment contains the active ingredient being studied.
- **Edema (Follicular Edema)**—An accumulation of an excessive amount of watery fluid in cells, tissues or serous cavities; redness.
- **Efficacy**—Power or capacity to produce a desired effect; effectiveness.
- **Electrologist**—A person who performs electrolysis.
- **Endocrinologist**—A physician who specializes in the endocrine system (glands and hormones). *Pediatric Endocrinologist* treats young patients.
- **Enzyme**—A protein which causes or speeds a specific reaction.
- **Epidermis**—The thin, protective outermost layer of skin.
- **Epithelial Cells**—The closely packed cells forming the epithelium.
- **Erythema**—Redness of skin.
- **Estrogen**—Hormone produced primarily in women that contributes to the development of secondary sex characteristics and cyclic changes such as menstruation and pregnancy.
- **Ethnicity**—Ethnic character, background or affiliation.
- **Etiology**—The study of causes or origins.
- **Exogenous**—Derived or developed from outside the body; originating externally.
- **External Root Sheath (ERS)**—One of two outer layers of the hair root; the ERS is the "lining" of the follicle wall and is continuous with the epidermis.
- **Familial**—Occurring or tending to occur among members of a family, usually by heredity.
- **FDA**—Food and Drug Administration.
- **Fertility**—The condition, quality or degree of being fertile.
- **Fitzpatrick Skin Type**—Measures skin tone and darkness by measuring the concentrations of melanin, hemoglobin and skin reflection properties.
- **Flush**—To turn red, as from fever, embarrassment or strong emotion; blush.
- **Follicle**—The tubular epithelial sheath that surrounds the lower part of the hair shaft. Hair follicles exist all over the body, with the exception of the palms, soles and mucous membranes. Hair follicles extend from the epidermal surface to deep into the dermis.

- **Follicular Bulb**—The deepest part of the follicle comprised of the combined germinal matrix and papilla.
- **Folliculitis**—An inflammation of the hair follicle; may include a pocket of pus (similar to acne).
- **Freckles**—Small brownish spot on the skin, often turning darker or increasing in number upon exposure to the sun.
- **Frustrated**—Discouraged, baffled, annoyed.
- **Gender Dysphoria**—Gender dysphoria, also known as "gender identity disorder," is a medical term for anxiety, confusion or discomfort about birth gender. Those who feel they have been born into the wrong gender are often aware that there is "something wrong" early in childhood. Because society places great emphasis on sexual and gender classification and on gender-appropriate behavior, such children will feel very different from their peers and uncertain about their identity.
- **Genetics**—The branch of biology that deals with heredity, especially the mechanisms of hereditary transmission and the variation of inherited characteristics among similar or related organisms.
- **Germal Matrix**—The growth zone in a hair follicle where hair is produced.
- **Glands**—Any organ or tissue that releases a substance used elsewhere in the body.
- **Gonadotrophin**—Any of a group of hormones secreted by the pituitary which stimulate the activity of the gonads.
- **Hair Bulb**—The bottom, rounded end of a hair follicle and site of hair productions.
- **Hair Root**—The part of the hair embedded in the skin.
- **Hair Shaft**—The portion of a hair external to the outer layer of the skin.
- **Hemoglobin**—The iron-containing respiratory pigment in red blood cells of vertebrates, consisting of about 6 percent heme and 94 percent globin.
- **Hereditary**—Transmitted or capable of being transmitted genetically from parent to offspring.
- **Hirsutism**—Excessive growth of terminal hair in androgen-dependent areas of a woman's body where terminal hair is not normally found, including the face, neck, chest and inner thighs.
- **Hormones**—A substance, usually a peptide or steroid, produced by one tissue and conveyed by the bloodstream to another to effect physiological activity, such as growth or metabolism.
- **Hyper-Pigmentation**—Excess pigmentation, especially of the skin.
- **Hyperandrogenism**—Increased levels of male hormone production in women.
- **Hypersecretion—Morbid or excessive secretion.**

- **Hyperthyroidism**—Pathologically excessive production of thyroid hormones.

- **Hypo-Pigmentation**—Diminished pigmentation, especially of the skin.

- **Hypodermis**—An epidermal layer of cells that secretes an overlying chitinous cuticle, as in arthropods. Also called subcutaneous tissue or subcutis, the fatty bottom layer of the skin that lies beneath the dermis and acts as an insulator and shock absorber. These tissues also store energy in the form of calories as a reserve nutritional source.

- **Iatrogenic**—Induced in a patient by a physician's activity, manner or therapy. Used especially of an infection or other complication of treatment.

- **Idiopathic**—Of, relating to, or designating a disease having no known cause.

- **Ineffective**—Not producing an intended effect; ineffectual: *an ineffective plea.*

- **Ingrown Hair**—This is when a hair curls back into the skin, and is often a result of plucking, shaving or waxing.

- **Inheritability**—Having the capacity to be inherited.

- **Inhibitor**—A substance that restrains or retards physiological, chemical or enzymatic action.

- **Insecure**—Not sure or certain; doubtful.

- **Insignificant**—Lacking in importance; trivial.

- **Insulin**—A polypeptide hormone secreted by the islets of Langerhans and functioning in the regulation of the metabolism of carbohydrates and fats, especially the conversion of glucose to glycogen, which lowers the blood glucose level.

- **Insulin Resistance**—In medicine, **insulin resistance** denotes a decompensation of glucose homeostasis where the tissues appear to be less responsive to insulin. Occurs when our cells stop responding to the insulin our pancreas makes. Too much insulin can actually cause hirsutism.

- **Internal Root Sheath (IRS)**—Soft keratin sheath derived from matrix cells covering the deepest half of the hair.

- **Investigation**—The act or process of investigating.

- **Irreversible**—Impossible to reverse.

- **Isotretinoin**—A synthetic retinoid, $C_{20}H_{28}O_2$, that inhibits sebaceous gland secretion and is used in the treatment of severe forms of acne.

- **Keloids**—A red, raised formation of fibrous scar tissue caused by excessive tissue repair in response to trauma or surgical incision.

- **Keratin**—Protein found in hair, nails and outer layers of skin. Keratin technically means "dead." For instance, if you cut the hair shaft you will not affect the hair's ability to continue to grow.

- **Keratinization**—The process of keratin production by keratinocyte cells.
- **Keratinocytes**—Cells that produce keratin.
- **Keratosis**—Excessive growth of horny tissue of the skin.
- **Knowledge**—The state or fact of knowing.
- **Laser**—A device that emits a beam of electromagnetic radiation. Often used in medical treatments such as hair removal.
- **Matrix**—The formative cells or tissue of a fingernail, toenail or tooth.
- **Medical Director**—In the United States, a **medical director** is typically a board-certified physician who is responsible for providing recommendations to EMS agencies. The medical director may also assist the agency in extending its scope of practice.
- **Medulla**—The inner core of certain organs or body structures, such as the marrow of bone.
- **Melanin Melanocytes**—Specialized epithelial cells that synthesize the melanin (pigment), which determines hair and skin color.
- **Mena**—A thin line of dark hair on the upper abdomen.
- **Menopause**—The period marked by the natural and permanent cessation of menstruation, occurring usually between the ages of 45 and 55.
- **Metabolite**—A metabolite is any substance produced or used during metabolism (digestion). In drug use, the term usually refers to the end product that remains after metabolism.
- **Minoxidil**—A vasodilator, $C_9H_{15}N_5O$, administered orally for the treatment of hypertension and used topically to promote the regrowth of hair in male pattern baldness.
- **Modalities**—Learning modalities are the sensory channels or pathways through which individuals give, receive and store information. Perception, memory and sensation comprise the concept of modality. The modalities or senses include visual, auditory, tactile/kinesthetic, smell and taste.
- **Monstrous**—Shockingly hideous or frightful.
- **Mortified**—Causing or experiencing shame, humiliation or wounded pride; humiliated.
- **MRI**—The use of a nuclear magnetic resonance spectrometer to produce electronic images of specific atoms and molecular structures in solids, especially human cells, tissues and organs.
- **Nationalities**—The status of belonging to a particular nation by origin, birth or naturalization.
- **NDA (New Drug Application)**—New drug application is required before someone can introduce a yet-unapproved drug on the market. There are several stages of this procedure.

- **Obesity**—The condition of being obese; increased body weight caused by excessive accumulation of fat.
- **Oestrogen**—Any of several steroid hormones produced chiefly by the ovaries and responsible for promoting estrus and the development and maintenance of female secondary sex characteristics.
- **Oligomenorrheic**—Abnormally light or infrequent menstruation
- **Oppressed**—To keep down by severe and unjust use of force or authority.
- **Ornithine Decarboxylase**—An enzyme that causes the matrix keratinocytes to divide.
- **Outcast**—One that has been excluded from a society or system.
- **Ovarian Tumors**—There are many kinds of ovarian tumors, and an ovarian tumor appears as a solid mass on an ultrasound. It is not as common as one might think. This is not to be confused with a cyst, which is fluid-filled and, most of the time, non-malignant. Although there are cysts that can turn into cancer, it is pretty rare for them to do so.
- **Papilla (Connective Tissue or Dermal Papilla)**—A small bit of dermal tissue that protrudes into the bottom of the hair bulb. The papilla contains a knot of capillaries that provide nutrients to the growing hair.
- **Pathophysiology**—Research that focuses on mechanisms of cellular growth and metabolism, and the role these processes play in human disease. It employs all of the scientific disciplines that are the basis of molecular medicine: physiology, molecular biology and genetics, cell biology, biochemistry, pharmacology, structural biology and immunology.
- **Perimenopause**—The period around the onset of menopause that is often marked by various physical signs (as hot flashes and menstrual irregularity).
- **Perseverance**—Steady persistence in adhering to a course of action, a belief or a purpose; steadfastness.
- **Phenotype**—The phenotype of an individual organism is either its total physical appearance and constitution or a specific manifestation of a trait, such as size or eye color, that varies between individuals.
- **Phenytoin**—Phenytoin sodium (marketed as Dilantin) is a commonly used antiepileptic. Phenytoin acts to damp the unwanted, runaway brain activity seen in seizure by reducing electrical conductance among brain cells.
- **Photosensitivity**—Sensitivity or responsiveness to light; an abnormally heightened response, especially of the skin, to sunlight or ultraviolet radiation, caused by certain disorders or chemicals and characterized by a toxic or allergic reaction.
- **Physical Gender**—Gender is a societal classification of people on the basis of physical and behavioral characteristics, such as genitals.

- **Physiologic**—Being in accord with or characteristic of the normal functioning of a living organism.

- **Pigment**—A substance, such as chlorophyll or melanin, that produces a characteristic color in plants or animals.

- **Pigmentary Changes**—Changes in the amount of melanin (colored substances) in the skin that cause the skin to darken or lighten.

- **PIH (Post Inflammatory Hyper-Pigmentation)**—Post-Inflammatory Hyper-Pigmentation (PIH) is a frequently encountered problem and represents the sequelae of various cutaneous disorders as well as therapeutic interventions.

- **Pituitary Gland**—A small oval endocrine gland attached to the base of the vertebrate brain and consisting of an anterior and a posterior lobe, the secretions of which control the other endocrine glands and influence growth, metabolism and maturation. Also called **hypophysis, pituitary body.**

- **Polyamines**—Any of a group of organic compounds, such as spermine and spermidine, composed of only carbon, nitrogen and hydrogen and containing two or more amino groups.

- **Polycystic Ovarian Syndrome (PCOS)**—An endocrine disorder, primarily in younger women, involving irregular menstrual periods and an excess of facial hair. The ovaries develop cysts and fail to release eggs; also known as SteinLeventhal Syndrome.

- **Port-Wine Stain**—A port-wine stain is a vascular (containing vessels) birthmark made of enlarged capillaries in the skin, which produce a reddish-purplish discoloration of the skin.

- **Predetermined**—Determined, decided or established in advance.

- **Progesterone**—A steroid hormone, $C_{21}H_{30}O_2$, secreted by the corpus luteum of the ovaries and by the placenta, that acts to prepare the uterus for implantation of the fertilized ovum, to maintain pregnancy, and to promote development of the mammary glands. **Prolactin** - A pituitary hormone that stimulates and maintains the secretion of milk.

- **Proliferation**—To grow or multiply by rapidly producing new tissue, parts, cells or offspring.

- **Protein**—Any of a group of complex organic macromolecules that contain carbon, hydrogen, oxygen, nitrogen and usually sulfur and are composed of one or more chains of amino acids. Proteins are fundamental components of all living cells and include many substances, such as enzymes, hormones and antibodies, which are necessary for the proper functioning of an organism. They are essential in the diet of animals for the growth and repair of tissue and can be obtained from foods such as meat, fish, eggs, milk and legumes.

- **Pseudofolliculitis Barbae ("razor bumps" or "razor burn")**—A common condition of the beard in men with curly hair. The hair grows back into the skin causing inflammation. Especially common in African Americans.

- **Purpura**—Purplish discoloration visible through the epidermis caused by hemorrhage into the tissues.
- **Race**—A local geographic or global human population distinguished as a more or less distinct group by genetically transmitted physical characteristics.
- **Radiology**—The branch of medicine that deals with the use of radioactive substances in diagnosis and treatment of disease.
- **Reduce**—To bring down, as in extent, amount or degree; diminish.
- **Repercussions**-An often indirect effect, influence or result that is produced by an event or action.
- **Resultant**—Issuing or following as a consequence or result.
- **Result**—To come about as a consequence.
- **Root Sheath**—The epidermal lining of a hair follicle.
- **Rosacea**—A chronic dermatitis of the face, especially of the nose and cheeks, characterized by a red or rosy coloration, caused by dilation of capillaries, and the appearance of acne-like pimples. Also called **acne rosacea**.
- **Sasquatch**—Large hairy humanoid creature said to live in wilderness areas of the United States and Canada [syn: Bigfoot].
- **Scarring**—A mark left on the skin after a surface injury or wound has healed.
- **Sebaceous (Oil) Gland**—Located at the upper portion of the hair follicle, sebaceous glands respond to testosterone, which causes them to enlarge. They manufacture sebum, which is oily and probably functions to moisturize the skin. Sebum drains into the hair follicle and then travels to the skin's surface.
- **Sebum**—The "skin oil" that lubricates our scalp and skin.
- **Secrete**—To release a substance used elsewhere in the body.
- **Self-Conscious**—Aware of oneself as an individual or of one's own being, actions or thoughts.
- **Self-Esteem**—Pride in oneself; self-respect.
- **Serum Levels**—The levels of the clear yellowish fluid obtained upon separating whole blood into its solid and liquid components after it has been allowed to clot.
- **Serum**—The clear yellowish fluid obtained upon separating whole blood into its solid and liquid components after it has been allowed to clot.
- **Sex Hormone-Binding Globulin (SHBG)**—A glycoprotein that binds to sex hormones, specifically testosterone and estradiol. Other

steroid hormones such as progesterone, cortisol and other corticosteroids are bound by transcortin.

- **Sexual Orientation**—The direction of one's sexual interest toward members of the same, opposite or both sexes.
- **Skin Tag**—An outgrowth of epidermal and dermal fibrovascular tissue. Also called *acrochordon, soft wart.*
- **Spironolactone**—A steroid derivative, $C_{24}H_{32}O_4S$, that blocks the action of aldosterone, used as a diuretic primarily in the treatment of hypertension.
- **Stimulation**—Arousal to activity or heightened action, as by spurring or goading; excitement.
- **Stimulus**—Something causing or regarded as causing a response.
- **Subcutaneous Tissue Layer**—This deeper layer of tissue lies beneath the dermis. The larger, deeper hair follicles and sweat glands originate here.
- **Subcutis**—See hypodermis.
- **Suppression**—Conscious exclusion of unacceptable desires, thoughts or memories from the mind.
- **Synergistic**—Producing or capable of producing synergy.
- **Synthesize**—To combine so as to form a new, complex product.
- **Taboo**—A ban or an inhibition resulting from social custom or emotional aversion.
- **Telangiectasia**—Chronic dilation of groups of capillaries causing elevated dark red blotches on the skin.
- **Telogen**—The resting phase in the hair growth cycle.
- **Terminal Hair**—Visible, dark, coarse hair that grows from birth. Terminal hair includes the hair on your head and eyebrows.
- **Testosterone**—An androgen that plays an important role in terminal hair growth.
- **Thermokinetic Selectivity**—Laser with TKS makes it possible for laser energy to "select" only hair follicles, while sparing surrounding skin from damage.
- **Thyroid**—A two-lobed endocrine gland found in all vertebrates, located in front of and on either side of the trachea in humans, and producing various hormones, such as triiodothyronine and calcitonin.
- **Tomography**—Any of several techniques for making detailed X-rays of a predetermined plane section of a solid object while blurring out the images of other planes.
- **Tormented**—Suffering great physical pain or mental anguish.
- **Transgenderists**—Transgenderists are persons who consistently live as members of the opposite gender either on a part- or full-time basis.

- **Transsexuals**—Those who wish to be considered by society as members of the opposite sex.
- **Treat**—To give medical aid to (someone): *treated many patients in the emergency room.*
- **Tretinoin**—A vitamin A derivative, $C_{20}H_{28}O_2$, which is a regulator substance in morphogenesis and functions in the growth and development of bone and the maintenance of epithelium.
- **Ugly**—Displeasing to the senses and morally revolting; "an ugly face."
- **Ultrasound**—The use of ultrasonic waves for diagnostic or therapeutic purposes, specifically to image an internal body structure, monitor a developing fetus, or generate localized deep heat to the tissues.
- **Vascular Lesion**—A vascular lesion is formed by abnormally large or numerous blood vessels located directly under the surface of the skin. These vessels may be visible through the skin or result in a red appearance of the skin. Spider veins (telangiectasia), shown to the right, are the most common vascular lesions.
- **Vellus Hair**—Fine hair present on the body after the Lanugo (downy) hair of the newborn is gone. These fine hairs cover most of the body into adulthood.
- **Venose**—Having noticeable veins or veinlike markings.
- **Virilizing**—Masculinisation.
- **Virilism**—The presence of male secondary sexual characteristics in a female.
- **Vital**—Of, relating to, or characteristic of life.
- **Wavelength**—The distance between one peak or crest of a wave of light, heat or other energy and the next corresponding peak or crest.

CHAPTER 21

RESOURCES AND REFERENCES

1) American College of Obstetricians and Gynecologists
P.O. Box 96920
Washington, DC 20090-6920
Phone: (202) 638-5577
www.acog.org

2) American Academy of Dermatology
P.O. Box 4014
Schaumburg, IL 60168-4014
Phone: (847) 330-0230
Toll-Free: (888) 462-3376
Fax: (847) 330-0050
www.aad.org

3) Creative Technologies (Meladine™), 1025 Executive Blvd.,
Suite 112 Chesapeake, VA 23320 info@creativeinc.biz

4) **HIRSUTISM**: A number of other sites on the Internet have
information about hirsutism. Information provided by the
National Institutes of Health, national medical societies, and some
other well-established organizations are often reliable sources of
information, although the frequency with which their information
is updated is variable.

- http://hirsutism.homestead.com/
- National Library of Medicine: www.nlm.nih.gov/medline plus/

5) **HORMONES:**
The Hormone Foundation: www.hormone.org
Natural Hormone Replacement (SottoPelle®): Dr Tutera

6) National Institute of Health (NIH), 9000 Rockville Pike,
Bethesda, MD 20892, 301-496-4000, www.nih.gov

7) Palomar Medical (IPL Medilux, Starlux etc.), 82 Cambridge
Street, Burlington, MA 01803   www.palmed.com

8) **PEDIATRIC ENDOCRINOLOGIST**:

Tala Dajani, M.D., M.P.H., Pediatric Endocrinologist, Internist, Phoenix Children's Hospital, 1919 East Thomas Rd, Phoenix, AZ 85016
ProCyte Corporation (Complex CU3 Intensive Tissue Repair), Redmond, VA 98052–www.procyte.com

9) **SHAVING:**

Does shaving stimulate hair growth/hypertrichosis? www.keratin.com/ah/ah018.shtml [keratin.com]—Includes references to a study done in the 1920s showing that there is no link between shaving and hair growth.

Structure and Function of Hair Follicles www.aad.org/education/hairfollicles.htm [American Academy of Dermatology]—Describes hair follicles and how they work.

Hair Myths www.heaven-earth.com/hairmyths/hairmyths.html—Points out that hair is dead, and cutting it has no effect on future growth, unless you damage the hair follicle, which is below the skin.

Top Ten Hair Myths www.hair-styles.org/top-10-hair-myths.html—Myth #1 is "Cutting your hair makes it stronger or grow faster." posted at 19:12:10 on 04/22/02 by Dennis <?memberid=1> - Category: Shaving <index.php?catid=2> headshaver.org/log/index.php?itemid=11
www.vanishmybumps.com/site/445529/page/127193?source=ga2
www.skinsite.com/info_pseudofolliculitis_barbae.htm
www.permanentchoice.com/Pages/electrolysis.htm

10) Skin Medica (Vaniqa), SkinMedica, Inc., 5909 Sea Lion Place, Ste H, Carlsbad, CA 92010 USA www.skinmedica.com

11) The Council Of Better Business Bureaus (BBB), 4200 Wilson Blvd., Suite 800, Arlington, VA 22203-1838, 1-703-276-0100, fax 1-703-525-8277, www.bbb.org **You can look up specific offices per state on this website*

12) **TRANSGENDER INFORMATION:**

• www.transgendercare.com

Douglas K. Ousterhout, M.D., D.D.S., 45 Castro Street, Suite 150, San Francisco, California 94114, (415) 626-2888, Copyright 1994 (1st Revision 1995) Douglas K. Ousterhout, M.D., D.D.S.
http://www.drbecky.com/dko.html

13) U.S. Food and Drug Administration (FDA), 5600 Fishers Lane, Rockville MD 20857-0001, 1-888-INFO-FDA (1-888-463-6332), www.fda.gov/default.htm

WEBSITES USED TO GATHER INFORMATION

Gold Therapy from: www.arthritis.ca/tips%20for%20living/understanding%20medications/disease%20modifying/gold%20therapy/default.asp?s=1
Women's Diaognostic Cyber,
http://www.wdxcyber.com/ninfer07.htm
http://www.blackwomenshealth.com/hirsutism.htm
http://www.bouldermedicalcenter.com/Articles/Hirsutism.htm
Where to get updated information about disorders:
www.uptodate.com
Menopause: www.fbhc.org/Patients/Modules/menopause.cfm
PCOS: www.pcossupport.org
CDLS: www.cdlsusa.org
Intelihealth.com
Teengrowth.com
The Hormone Foundation (www.hormone.org)
www.cdlsusa.org/about_cdls/faq.html#recognized
Patients.update.com

www.symposion.com/ijt/ijtc0405m.htm

www.intelihealth.com/IH/ihtIH/WSIHW000/9339/10144.html

www.accessexcellence.org/WN/SUA05/wolfman.html

www.mothernature.com/Library/Bookshelf/Books/16/99.cfm

en.wikipedia.org/wiki/Hypertrichosis

www.teengrowth.com/index.cfm?action=info_advice&ID_Advice=
28676

kidshealth.org/teen/your_body/skin_stuff/hair_removal.html

MORE RESOURCES

**I obtained a wealth of information for this book from Skin
Medica® (Vaniqa®). _The following resources are strictly from the
Skin Medica/Vaniqa information, charts, statistics etc._**

Hatch, R.; Rosenfield, R.S.; Kim, M.H.; Tredway, D. "Hirsutism:
Implications, etiology, and management." _Am J Obstet Gynecol_
1981; 140:815.

O'Driscoll, J.B.; Mamtora, H.; Higginson, J.; et al. "A prospective
study of the prevalence of clear-cut endocrine disorders and polycystic ovaries in 350 patients presenting with hirsutism or androgenic alopecia." _Clin Endocrinol_ 1994; 41:231.

Ferriman, D.; Gallwey, J.D. "Clinical assessment of body hair
growth in women." _J Clin Endocrinol Metab_ 1961; 21:1440.

Derksen, J.; Nagesser, S.K.; Meinders, A.E.; et al. "Identification of
virilizing adrenal tumors in hirsute women." _N Engl J Med_ 1994;
331:968.
Marieb, E.N. _Human Anatomy and Physiology._ 3rd ed.
Redwood City, California: Benjamin/Cummings; 1995.

Shai, A.; Maibach, H.I.; Baran, R. "Skin Structure." In: _Handbook
of Cosmetic SkinCare._ 1st ed. London, England: Martin Dunitz
Ltd.; 2001:5-17.

Ham, A.W.; Cormack, D.C. "The Integumentary System
(The Skin and Its Appendages)." In: _Histology._ 8th ed.
Philadelphia, PA; Toronto, Canada: J.B Lippincott Company;
1979:614-640.

Shai, A.; Maibach, H.I.; Baran, R. "Structure of Hair and Principles of Hair Care." In: *Handbook of Cosmetic Skin Care.* 1st ed. London, England: Martin Dunitz Ltd.; 2001:251-262.

Fitzpatrick et al (eds): *Dermatology in General Medicine.* 5th ed. New York, NY: McGraw-Hill; 1999.

Nippon Menard Cosmetics Co. Ltd.; 2001. www.menard.co.jp/english/. Accessed June 2004.

Data on File at Bristol Meyers Squibb 1999.

Shai, A.; Maibach, H.I.; Baran, R. "Methods for Temporary Removal of Hair." In: *Handbook of Cosmetic Skin Care.* 1st ed. London, England: Martin Dunitz Ltd.; 2001:282-292.

Azziz, R. "Advances in the evaluation and treatments of unwanted hair growth." *Contemporary OB/GYN* Feb 2002:2-10.

"Methods of hair removal: Prescription oral medications." www.hairfacts.com. Updated Dec 2001. Accessed June 2004.

Mayo Clinic Staff, Women's Health Center. "Polycystic ovary syndrome: treatment." www.mayoclinic.com. Updated Feb 2004. Accessed June 2004.

Jelovsek, F.R. "Facial hair growth after menopause." Woman's Diagnostic Cyber, www.wdxcyber.com. Updated June 2002. Accessed June 2004.

Huber, F.; Schrode, K.; Stazak, J.; et al. "Outcome of a quality-of-life assessment used in clinical trials for hirsute women treated with topical eflornithine 15 percent cream." Presented at the American

Laura M. Regan

Academy of Dermatology Annual Meeting, San Francisco, CA, March 11-14, 2000.

Balfour, J.A.; McClellan, K. "Topical eflornithine." Am J Clin Dermatol. 2001;2(3):197-201.

Shai, A.; Maibach, H.I.; Baran, R. "Permanent Hair Removal: Electrolysis—electric needle." In: Handbook of Cosmetic Skin Care. 1st ed. London, England: Martin Dunitz Ltd.; 2001:293-302.

Grekin, R.; Zachary, C. "A comparison between the Lyra Long-Pulsed Nd:YAG laser system and the Coherent LightSheer Diode laser system in the removal of hair." www.lasernews.net.V3. Accessed June 2004.

Littler, C.M. "Hair removal using an Nd:YAG laser system." Derm Clin 1999;17:401-430.

Battle, E.; Suthamjariya, K.; Alora, B.; Palli, K.; Anderson, R.R. "Very long-pulsed diode laser for hair removal on all skin types." Lasers Surg Med. 2000;12(Suppl):85.

Chui, C.T.; Grekin, R.C.; Le Boit, P.E.; Zachary, C.B. "Long-pulsed Nd:YAG for hair removal: early histological changes." 1999 LaserNews.net. The Journal: Vol 1 Issue 1, Jan 2000. www.lasernews.net. Accessed June 2004.

Rogachefsky, A.S.; Silapunt, S.; Goldberg, D.J. "Evaluation of a new super-long-pulsed 810 nm diode laser for the removal of unwanted hair: the concept of thermal damage time." Dermatol Surg. 2002;28:4l0-4l4.

Battle, E.F.; Hobbs, L.M. "Laser-assisted hair removal for darker skin types." Dermatol Ther. 2004;17(2):177-183.

Bashour, M. "Laser hair removal." www.emedicine.com Updated May 2002. Accessed June 2004.

"Laser hair removal." American Academy of Dermatology, Public Resources. www.aad.org/PressReleases. July 27, 2003. Accessed June 2004.

Tanzi, E.L.; Alster, T.S. "Long-pulsed 1064-nm Nd:YAG laser-assisted hair removal in all skin types." *Dermatol Surg.* 2004 Jan;30(l):13-17.

Bouzari, N.; Tabatabai, H.; Abbasi, Z.; Firooz, A.; Dowlati, Y. "Laser hair removal: comparison of long-pulsed Nd:YAG, long pulsed alexandrite, and long-pulsed diode lasers." *Dermatol Surg.* 2004 Apr;30(4 pt 1):498-502.

Galadari, I. "Comparative evaluation of different hair removal lasers in skin types IV, V, and VI." *Int J Dermatol.* 2003 Jan;42(l):68-70.

Hamzavi, I.; Tan, E.; Shapiro, J.; Lui, H. "Combined treatment with laser and topical eflornithine is more effective than laser treatment alone for removing unwanted facial hair—a placebo-controlled trial." Presented at the American Society of Laser Medicine and Surgery Annual Meeting, Anaheim, CA, 2003.

Smith, S.R.; Pacquadio, D.J.; Littler, C. "Eflornithine cream combined with laser therapy in the management of unwanted facial hair growth in women—a randomized trial." Presented at the American Association of Dermatologists Annual Meeting, San Francisco, CA, March 21-26, 2003.

ABOUT THE AUTHOR

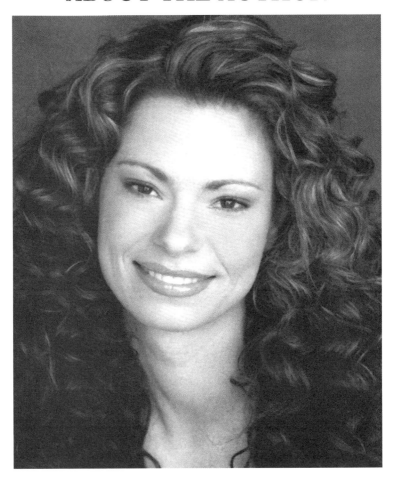

Laura M. Regan is the CEO/CFO of Divine Laser Hair Removal, Inc. and Divine Secrets Skincare, Inc. in Phoenix, Arizona. Certified as both an electrologist and medical laser technician, she has been formally trained in laser procedures, skincare treatments and products and intense pulsed light systems. Laura has also formulated an exclusive "combination therapy" for patients who have special needs due to hormonal imbalances. Laura and Divine Laser have appeared on numerous TV and radio shows including Good Evening Arizona.

FINAL NOTE

I was browsing through *Glamour* magazine and came across the below article. The article is a funny and ironic take on female "hairiness" from a male perspective. I wanted to share it with all of you as my final note because it summarizes the entire meaning behind my book...YOU'RE NOT ALONE in your "hair" struggle. Most people probably don't notice your "hairiness" or, they may completely accept it and even like it in some circumstances!

Hairy parts

Some men are obsessed with kind-of-hairy women and don't even know it; they just keep ending up with girlfriends who have big, dark eyebrows and thick, lush nether regions (yes, we guys have been known to discuss what you've got down there). While I admit to getting scared off by nipple hair occasionally, I have to say I was glad to see the trend in thick eyebrows come back in, and I don't need women to be perfectly smooth and hair free on the rest of her body either. After all, we're just slightly evolved animals. Sleeping with a fully waxed woman is like sleeping with a store-window mannequin. That may be hot for the few fetishists who lurk around Bloomingdale's, but the rest of us prefer warm-blooded mammals.

*The article was in the October 2006 edition of **Glamour** *magazine under Men, Sex & Love. The title of the article is: Body "flaws" you hate....but he loves, Guys think you're hot even if you think you're not, says Jake.*

Jake is a real guy, living single and writing in New York City. Send him your feedback at glamour.com/jake.